"This book has the potenti[al...]
leading expert on the topic o[f...]
a masterful job of applying r[...]
format. This journal could be [used...] therapy,
as a comprehensive tool that includes the core components to soothe emotional pain, build coping skills, and find hope."

—**Scott Waltman, PsyD, ABPP**, president-elect of both the Academy of Cognitive and Behavioral Therapies, and the International Association of CBT; and lead author of *The Stoicism Workbook*

"Kathryn Hope Gordon's guided journal is a compassionate, practical resource for those facing mental health challenges. With evidence-based tools and gentle prompts, it empowers readers to navigate crises, nurture self-compassion, and build hope. Gordon's expertise as a therapist and researcher shines, making this a valuable companion for anyone seeking safety, connection, and healing."

—**Ted Bender, PhD, MBA**, chief operating officer of ABA Centers

"*The Suicidal Thoughts Guided Journal* is an accessible, step-by-step, nonjudgmental method to handle suicidality. Written in warm, empathic, and earnest language, Kathryn Hope Gordon has put together a complete, science-based, aide-de-camp for clinicians, their clients, and even family members of people affected by suicidality. The activities and exercises in the journal are explained in everyday terms that will help individuals navigate current suicidal crises and build a hopeful life plan for the future."

—**Leonardo Bobadilla, PhD**, associate professor of psychology at Pacific University

"This wonderful, immediately useful journal will save lives. The prompts guide readers struggling with suicidal thoughts toward authentic expression, perspective taking, and actionable steps to strengthen their connections to life. I'm so grateful to Kathryn Hope Gordon for creating such an outstanding resource that will bring hope to countless people."

—**Joel Minden, PhD**, psychologist, and author of *Show Your Anxiety Who's Boss*

"Kathryn Hope Gordon beautifully balances the provision of science-based information and empirically supported techniques with a warm and compassionate style of delivery. Her guidance does not read like a set of instructions; rather, working through this book feels more like having a conversation with a caring and knowledgeable friend. Readers will find that the exercises facilitate healing while her words inspire hope."

—**Yessenia Castro, PhD**, associate professor and associate dean for doctoral education n the Steve Hicks School of Social Work at The University of Texas at Austin

"From the very first page, this guided journal creates a sense of warmth, safety, and validation. Through compassionate writing and practical exercises, it provides readers with strategies to navigate suicidal thoughts and tools to build a more hopeful future. Thoughtfully designed, it feels less like a clinical workbook and more like a supportive companion, offering reassurance and actionable steps to those who need it most."

—**April R. Smith, PhD**, alumni professor of psychological sciences at Auburn University, and director of the Research on Eating Disorders and Suicidality Laboratory

"This is an excellent resource for those navigating tough moments and heavy hearts. It provides meaningful, practical, approachable exercises that are evidence-based and compassionate—and are a toolkit to reduce overwhelm. These prompts and exercises that Kathryn Hope Gordon has written are a guide to navigating difficult experiences, and can be an entry point or supplement to professional help."

—**Jessica B. Stern**, clinical psychologist, consultant, speaker, CEO of Three Lemons LLC, and assistant professor of psychiatry at NYU Langone Health

The

Suicidal Thoughts
Guided Journal

CBT PRACTICES *to*
SOOTHE EMOTIONAL PAIN,
BUILD COPING SKILLS,
and FIND HOPE

KATHRYN HOPE GORDON, PhD

New Harbinger Publications, Inc.

Publisher's Note

This publication is designed to provide accurate and authoritative information in regard to the subject matter covered. It is sold with the understanding that the publisher is not engaged in rendering psychological, financial, legal, or other professional services. If expert assistance or counseling is needed, the services of a competent professional should be sought.

INSTANT HELP, the Clock Logo, and NEW HARBINGER are trademarks of New Harbinger Publications, Inc.

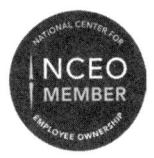

New Harbinger Publications is an employee-owned company.

Copyright © 2025 by Kathryn Hope Gordon

                    Instant Help Books
                    An imprint of New Harbinger Publications, Inc.
                    5720 Shattuck Avenue
                    Oakland, CA 94609
                    www.newharbinger.com

All Rights Reserved

Cover design by Amy Shoup

Interior design by Tom Comitta

Illustrations by Alyse Ruriani

Acquired by Ryan Buresh

Edited by Iris van de Pavert

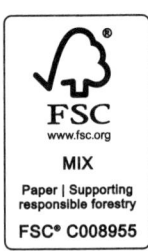

Printed in the United States of America

27   26   25

10   9   8   7   6   5   4   3   2   1   First Printing

*To Keith, Lyla, Graham, Mary (Mom), Les (Dad),
Annie, and Linda, I love you endlessly.*

*To all who suffer with suicidal thoughts,
I hope you find support in these words.
I wrote them for you.*

CONTENTS

Crisis Phone & Text Lines — ix
Foreword — xi
Introduction — 1

PART 1: COPE WITH CRISES — 5

Know Your Warning Signs — 6
Seek Support — 10
Increase Your Safety — 15
Your Reasons for Living — 18
Decrease Emotional Intensity — 21
Make a Crisis Plan — 27

PART 2: SOOTHE EMOTIONAL PAIN — 31

Uncover Causes and Context — 32
True Self-Care — 34
Problem-Solve — 38
Analyze Painful Thoughts — 43
Reframe Painful Thoughts — 53

PART 3: NURTURE SELF-COMPASSION — 61

Experiences of Discrimination — 65
Self-Validation — 69
Your Sources of Strength — 71
What Would You Tell a Friend? — 74

Show Yourself Kindness 77
Cultivate Acceptance 81

PART 4: BUILD HOPE — 89

Seek Help 94
Find Optimism 99
Change Perspective 103
Attend to Emotions 108
Make a Hope Box 115

PART 5: CONNECT WITH PEOPLE — 117

Strengthen Connections 118
Explore Emotional Safety 123
You Belong 127
You Are Not a Burden 133

PART 6: MAKE MEANING — 137

Identify Your Values 139
Find Meaning in Actions and Experiences 140
Find Meaning in Relationships 143
Find Meaning in Suffering 145
Make a Meaning Collage 147

Conclusion 149

Additional Resources 154

Acknowledgments 157

References 159

CRISIS PHONE & TEXT LINES

United States

The *988 Suicide & Crisis Lifeline* is free and available 24/7 to anyone who reaches out with suicidal thoughts or other emotional distress. When you contact them, a trained crisis counselor will provide confidential support.

Call: 988
Website: http://www.988lifeline.org

Around the World

The International Association for Suicide Prevention created a *Suicidal Crisis Support* directory. You can search for helplines in your country through their website: http://www.iasp.info/suicidalthoughts.

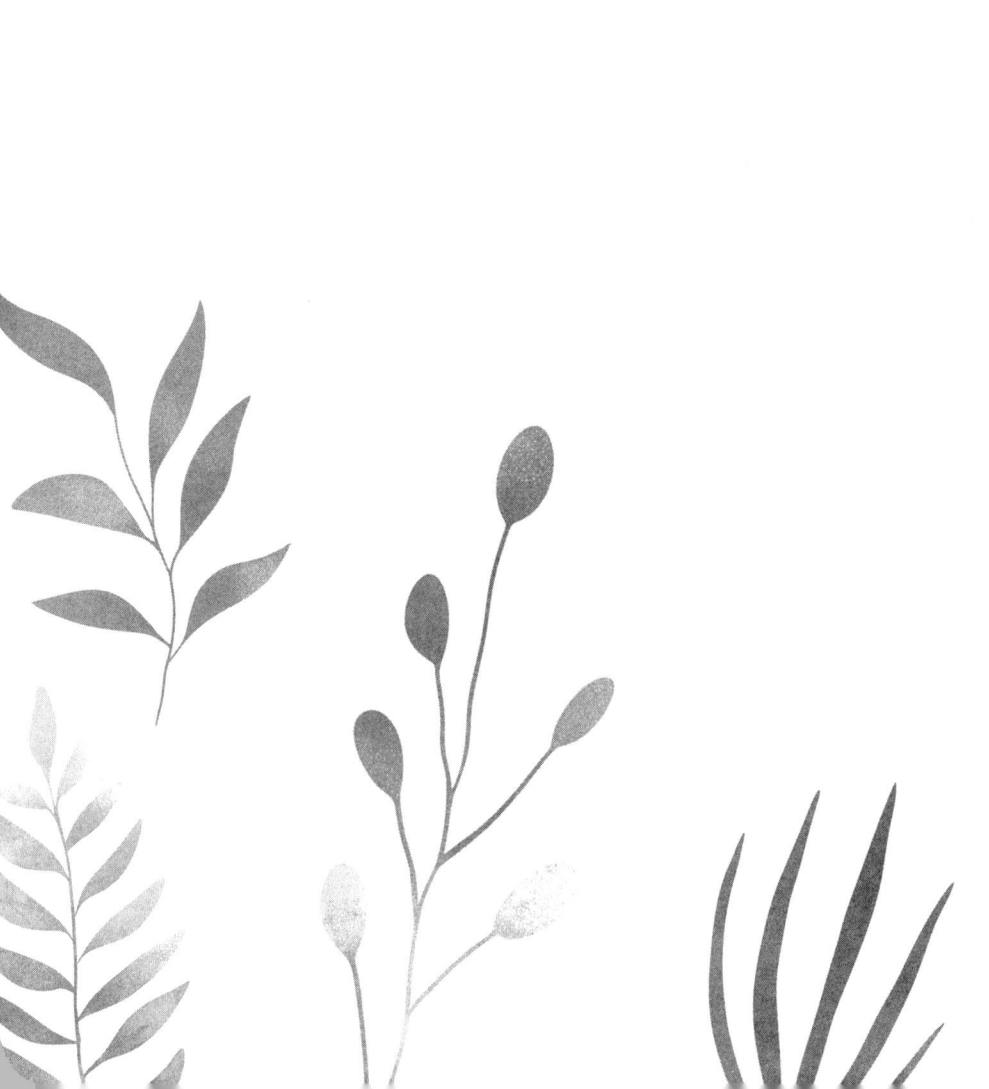

FOREWORD

According to the National Survey on Drug Use and Health, an estimated 12.8 million adults in the US had serious suicidal thoughts in 2023–that means that almost 5% of the American adult population were in such a state of excruciating pain that they were considering ending their lives. In 2019, Dr. David Jobes and I wrote that many people struggling with suicidal thoughts do so in silent misery; therefore, suicidal thoughts must become an essential target of intervention. Dr. Gordon's guided journal does exactly that. Drawing from her clinical and scientific expertise, her book addresses suicidal thoughts directly and provides practical tools to alleviate them.

My research group recently contended that people enter a liminal psychological state preceding suicide that arises from an undermined sense of agency–an ability to act and influence one's life. We asserted that this diminished sense of agency produces an uncannily painful, almost indescribable mind state, in which people are conscious of moment-to-moment experiences but feel lifeless, unable to sense their own existence. Tragic, jarring, grave, and profound stuff, I know. All the more reason to ensure that agency thrives.

This is just one of the reasons I am excited for Dr. Gordon's book; its raison d'être is the cultivation of hope. Hope and agency overlap considerably; they leverage and scaffold one another. Hope is the antidote to feeling trapped in a state of suffering. In addition to hope, Dr. Gordon's book focuses on building agency through several other skills, such as problem solving, support seeking, meaning-making, self-compassion, thought reframing, and effectively navigating life's hardships.

In late 2020, during the relatively early months of a global pandemic, I wrote in the foreword of Dr. Gordon's Suicidal Thoughts Workbook, "… the current book is hopeful. How can that be? For one thing, the book's author has a hopeful disposition, a fact to which I can attest having known her for close to 20 years, and a fact which animates the pages that follow. Her hopefulness is not hollow but rather is hard-won through many years of clinical experience, and that is apparent in these pages as well." I have now known her for well over 20 years, and would add of her and of her book, that she and it are down-to-earth and relatable. These attributes and features make for an optimistic, feasible, and effective way forward for those in the throes of suicidal crises.

Dr. Gordon's recommendations in this book represent real gains in the treatment of suicidal thoughts. Paired with her relatable approach, this compassionate, practical book contributes to the important endeavor of disseminating useful mental health interventions to as many people as possible.

—Thomas Ellis Joiner, Jr., PhD

INTRODUCTION

Welcome!

I'm so glad you're here. Thank you for seeking help for your suicidal thoughts. I know how hard it is to work on your mental health when you're suffering, especially if you've been struggling for a long time. I appreciate your openness to exploring the tools in this journal. My hope is that this journal empowers you with ways to feel better as you face the challenges in your life. You are worthy of support.

> *I promise that your life matters so much.*
> *The world is better with you in it,*
> *even if it doesn't feel like it right now.*

That's why I want to make sure you're safe. If you're currently having suicidal thoughts, please stop reading this journal and contact one of the crisis lines on the previous page (call 988 in the United States). Once you're safe, you can return to this journal.

A Space for You

If you're safe right now and ready to read on, I want you to know that this journal is a space just for you. You can express yourself without judgment, reflect on your experiences, and learn skills designed to ease the painful parts of life while making your life more enjoyable and meaningful. You deserve compassion as you process your experiences, and I hope you find that here.

The Power of Journaling

Research points to the following as related to suicide risk (in addition to other factors): pain that is emotional, psychological, or physical, hopelessness, feeling alone or like you don't belong, isolation, feeling like a burden, feeling disconnected from life (like there are no reasons for living or life lacks meaning), and access to lethal suicide methods (e.g., Klonsky et al. 2021; O'Connor 2022; Van Orden et al. 2010). As a therapist, I've observed the power of journaling as a pathway to healing for many of my patients as they face these kinds of hardships.

In this journal, you will learn ways to address each of the factors above. For example, you'll gain greater insight into how your thoughts, feelings, and behaviors influence your well-being and learn effective coping strategies to improve your mental health and safety. Each skill and prompt in this journal was carefully selected from my decades of experience as a therapist and suicide researcher. In addition to helping my patients, these tools help me in my own life. They can help you too.

How to Use This Guided Journal

Sometimes, people feel stuck when they start writing. They aren't sure what to say or if what they're writing is useful. That inspired me to create a guided journal. Like traditional journals, each entry has an open space for your thoughts, feelings, and anything else that comes to mind. The guided part means that you'll also find prompts and skills to try while journaling.

I've noticed that my patients also have a tough time finding the time to journal. Many of us are busy, feel too tired, or have difficulty focusing when we're hurting. That's why I aimed to make each entry take no longer than 5–15 minutes to complete. You don't have to make major changes at a rapid pace to start feeling better. You can take small steps at a comfortable pace. These ripples tend to add up over time and turn into impactful changes.

I recommend that you set a realistic goal for writing in this journal. For some people, this may be as frequent as fifteen minutes or more per day. For others, it may be more realistic to write in the journal once per week. You're more likely to experience benefits from a consistent pattern of working on your mental health, whatever that looks like for you.

You may find this journal to be a helpful addition to therapy, which I recommend to anyone who is struggling. Professional support can be quite useful for navigating painful suicidal thoughts. I also know that therapy can be hard to access for different reasons (like financial, wait lists, or a desire for a self-help approach). You can also begin using this journal on your own outside of therapy. First and foremost, the journal is here to help you in whatever way you best see fit. I've written it with adults in mind and recommend seeking out other resources if you are a child or teen (for example, *Overcoming Suicidal Thoughts for Teens*, Pettit and Hill 2022).

Use What's Helpful, Discard What Isn't

I recommend starting with "Part 1: Cope with Crises" because crisis and safety plans are especially helpful for preventing suicide in people with suicidal thoughts (e.g., Rogers et al. 2022; Stanley et al. 2018). After completing that section, please feel free to write in the guided journal in order or skip around to different parts that speak to your current needs. I aimed to offer a variety of options so you can find tools and solutions that resonate with you. Please return to the tools you find most useful as many times as you need them. Most skills become stronger and more effective with repeated practice.

However, you may also find yourself trying a skill and disliking it or finding it unhelpful. That doesn't mean anything is wrong with you. It's not your fault. We all have different strategies that work best for us and those that aren't a good match for our preferences or circumstances. Please stop using anything in this journal that doesn't serve you. In fact, if at any time you feel like your suicidal thoughts are worsening while writing in this journal, *please stop that exercise or prompt right away*. Reach out to a crisis line (like 988 in the United States) any time that your suicidal thoughts become more severe.

Give Yourself Grace

There's no wrong way to use this journal. If you come across setbacks or times where you're less consistent with writing in it, please be gentle with yourself. You're going through a lot right now. The world can be a hard place, and you may be facing challenges that are getting in the way. When you're ready, you can return to the journal. I'm rooting for you and wishing you the very best as you work on your mental health.

You are worthy of compassion, support, and joy.

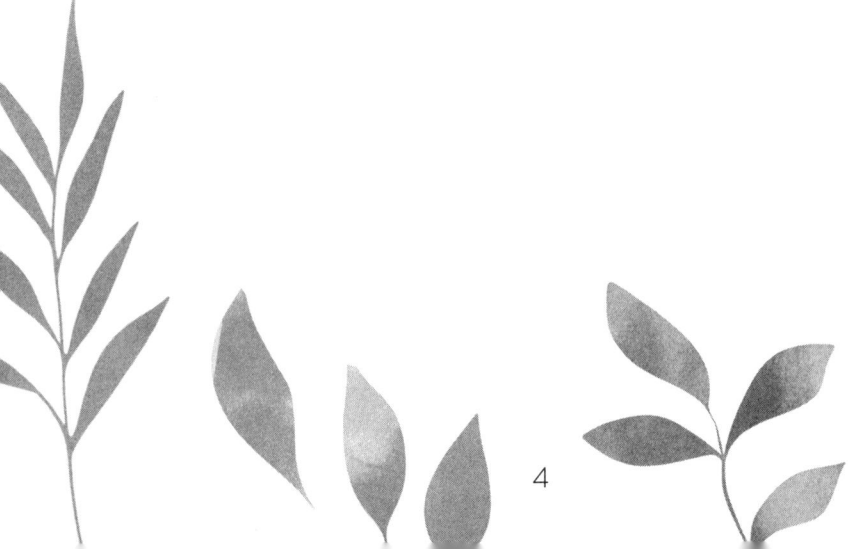

Part 1

COPE WITH CRISES

When you're in the middle of a crisis, it's hard to come up with ways to get help and stay safe. That's why in this first section of the journal, we'll work together to create an emergency plan you can use in those moments. We'll find ways to identify your warning signs, seek support, increase safety, remember your reasons for living, and ease emotional intensity. Then, we'll pull it all together into a personalized one-page crisis plan.

Know Your Warning Signs

Please find a space for yourself where you feel comfortable writing. Now, take some even breaths and reflect on times when you've experienced a suicidal crisis. While it's helpful to recall past crises so you can identify the warning signs of a future crisis, they can be painful to think about. Go at your own pace and take breaks as you need them. When you're ready, write about the times that come to mind. You don't have to include every detail, but take time to pay attention to:

- the events that led up to the crisis or crises
- how your body felt
- the thoughts that went through your mind
- any signs other people might be able to see from the outside.

You can write this in paragraph or list form—whatever feels most useful for you.

I'm so glad that you made it through those crises and that you're still with us.

What did it feel like to look back on those times? Share your feelings in the space below.

Now that you've looked back on past crises, what warning signs do you see? I've listed some possibilities below. Please add any warning signs that don't appear on the list:

- stress (for instance, loss of a loved one, housing, health, legal, or financial problems, chronic pain, employment issues, conflicts, trauma, mental health problems, the end of a relationship)
- agitation
- self-hatred
- shame
- social withdrawal or isolation
- making suicide plans
- preparing methods for suicide
- hygiene worsening
- humiliation
- changes in substance use
- changes in eating
- changes in sleeping (like increased insomnia or nightmares)
- mood changes
- feeling like you have no purpose in life
- feeling trapped
- acting impulsively or recklessly
- feeling like a burden
- imagining suicide or death
- _____
- _____
- _____
- _____
- _____

If you recognize a stressor; any changes in your sleep, mood, or eating; or impulsive or reckless behavior, please be specific in your journaling. For instance, specify what changed in your substance use or what you did when you acted impulsively.

Which items on the list did you recognize? Any you've added yourself?

It may hurt to think about past crises, but I hope you came away from the exercise with a better understanding of your warning signs. That will make it easier to spot an oncoming crisis in the future. Please take a moment to feel proud of yourself for working through this process, even though it's hard.

Seek Support

In most emergency situations, we do much better with support from others, and suicidal crises are no different. Now that we've figured out some of the warning signs, let's take some time to think about who you can count on for help.

Reflect on the people in your life who support you most. Have any of them helped you during past crises? If so, how?

If you had trouble coming up with people who you can count on, you're not alone. Part 5 of the journal focuses on tools for increasing supportive connections with people.

Please take a few moments to write about how you feel right now after writing about people's past responses to your suicidal crises.

Let's turn your journal reflections into more specific crisis response plans by listing people by name along with the way they can best help you during a crisis. If you have trouble thinking of people, consider the following as possibilities: relatives, partners, friends, coworkers, neighbors, mental health professionals, medical professionals, people from groups you belong to (for instance, spiritual communities, clubs, or organizations), clergy, mentors, peers, coaches, and suicide crisis lines.

Try to think of at least one person or resource for each category below if you can. It's okay to put the same person in multiple categories.

Who lifts your spirits?

_____

_____

_____

Whom can you share your feelings with?

_____

_____

_____

Who can help you with your coping or problem-solving skills?

_____

_____

_____

Who can keep you company when you're lonely?

Who can help you stay physically safe?

I hope you found it beneficial to name supportive people or resources you can turn to during a crisis. No one should have to go through tough times alone. If you have a hard time expressing you need help, you may want to try saying one of the lines below:

- *I feel really down right now. Can I talk to you about it?*
- *I'm struggling and don't know what to do. Do you have ideas about how I can get help?*
- *I'm having thoughts about suicide and feeling scared and lonely. Can we meet up or talk on the phone?*

What are some other ways you can ask for support?

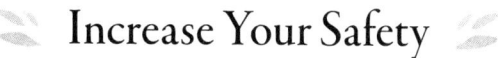 Increase Your Safety

Suicidal thoughts tend to fluctuate over time. Even intense suicidal thoughts can diminish within hours of their onset (Coppersmith et al. 2023). If you reduce access to self-harm methods during strong suicidal urges, you will lower your risk for a suicide attempt. The more time that passes without access to a self-harm method, the more likely it is that the suicidal thought will lessen in strength without you getting hurt.

How can you make your environment safer when you're in a crisis? Are there any obstacles that could get in the way? How can you address these obstacles?

Did you come up with some ideas for keeping yourself safe during suicidal crises? If so, that's wonderful. You just took some important steps toward self-protection. If not, that's understandable. You may have had only a little practice or maybe never thought about crises this way before. I've created a guide below to help you through this potentially life-saving exercise.

Do you have any guns in your home?

- ☐ Yes.
- ☐ No.

Which of the following ways can you increase safety when you're in a crisis?

- ☐ Store the gun(s) outside of your home (like a trusted person's house who is okay with helping).
- ☐ Store the bullets separate from the gun(s).
- ☐ Use a lockbox or gun safe.
- ☐ Use a gun lock.
- ☐ Other ways: _____

Are there other potential self-harm methods in your home that you could reduce access to during a crisis (like medications or sharps)? How can you restrict access to these methods when you're in a crisis? If you're not sure, consider asking a medical or mental health professional, a friend, or another person for ideas and suggestions. You can also contact a crisis line (for instance, 988) for help with making your environment safer and for help with addressing any obstacles you've identified.

Write about other ways to increase safety here:

Your Reasons for Living

When you're feeling suicidal, your mind may be like a magnet attracting thoughts about reasons for dying. Meanwhile, your reasons for living may feel more distant. One helpful strategy is to make a reasons for living list to reference during times of crisis. If you have trouble thinking of ideas, consider your answers to the following questions:

What keeps you going? What do you look forward to? Who do you want to keep spending time with? What would you miss out on if you weren't alive? Who do you feel most connected to in your life? What do you feel most strongly about in your life?

How are you feeling after journaling about your reasons for living? I hope you found it clarifying and insightful. However, you might feel stuck. That's okay too. I've created a guide for further reflection on your reasons for living. Circle any reason that is true for you and, importantly, add any that are missing from the list. No reason for living is too trivial or small—include whatever tethers you to life.

My reason(s) for living are:

- I want to spend more time with my loved ones.
- I don't want my loved ones to feel sad.
- I want to see my child(ren) grow up.
- I have religious or spiritual reasons for wanting to live.
- I want to take care of my pet(s).
- I'm afraid to die.
- I don't want to miss out on good times in the future.
- My life might improve.
- I want to make the world a better place.
- I'm excited about future plans.
- I feel bad now, but I might feel better in the future.
- I find joy in my interests and hobbies.
- My life has meaning.
- If I can get through this, I can help others who are struggling.
- I have more I want to accomplish in my life.
- Even when I'm in pain, I still have joyful moments.
-
-
-
-

Now that you've had time to think about your reasons for living, which ones are the most important?

Why are those your most important reasons for living?

You did a fantastic job reflecting on your reasons for living. Shining a spotlight on these reasons now will help you to remember them more easily later if you're in a crisis. One way to amplify your list is to take what you've written and get creative. You can draw, sketch, make a collage of pictures, make music, write a poem—whatever feels most helpful for you. Then, you can place your creation somewhere you will see it regularly. Consider sharing it with loved ones so they can better understand you. They can remind you of your reasons for living too.

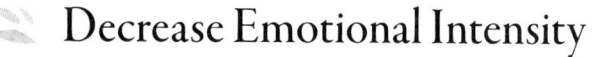 # Decrease Emotional Intensity

When you have suicidal thoughts, what emotions do you tend to experience? What does your body feel like? What types of thoughts are running through your head?

If you raise your awareness about these emotions, feelings, and thoughts here, you'll be ready for the next step: identifying strategies to navigate them.

I appreciate you reflecting on your emotions, feelings, and thoughts while in past crises. It's hard to recall those times, but I hope you find it worth it and feel more prepared for the future.

What types of coping have you used to decrease the intensity of your suicidal thoughts and feelings in the past? Which ones were most helpful? Which were less helpful? Why do you think those particular coping skills were effective or ineffective for you?

Were you able to identify some useful coping strategies during suicidal crises? If so, that's great!

However, if you struggled to think of effective coping strategies, that's okay too. It can be hard to figure this out.

As I mentioned in the beginning of the book, all of us find certain tools work better for us than others. If any of them lack impact or make you feel worse, please stop using them. There's a certain amount of trial and error that we all endure in the search for our favorite tools. It's a necessary part of the path to ultimately finding what will help you the most. Please treat yourself with warmth and patience as you stick with this process.

As a starting point, I've observed that the intensity of thoughts, emotions, and feelings during suicidal crises tends to decrease for patients when they engage in activities that:

- absorb a lot of attention
- influence them physically in a positive way
- evoke positive feelings.

I've listed some activities with those components below. Circle the ones you would like to try or that you think would be helpful for decreasing emotional intensity during suicidal crises. Importantly, please add your own ideas to the list too:

- Read, watch, or listen to a captivating or comforting movie, book, TV show, or podcast episode.
- Play video, computer, or phone games.
- Work on a home improvement project.
- Build something.
- Knit or crochet.
- Paint nails.
- Do a puzzle.
- Play a tabletop game.

- Talk with a friend.
- Go for a walk.
- Cuddle with a pet or person.
- Take a shower or bath.
- Take a nap.
- Listen to soothing music.
- Find a change of scenery.
- Drink hot tea.
- Play with a fidget toy.
- Stretch.
- Play a sport.
- Hug a loved one.
- Browse books at a store or library.
- Do a relaxation exercise.
- Look at funny pictures or memes.
- Look at pictures of things or places that make you happy.
- Dance or sing.
- Pray or meditate.
- Sit outside.
- Wrap yourself in a blanket.
- Play an instrument.
- Write or read a poem.
- _____
- _____
- _____
- _____
- _____
- _____

After working through that list of activities to reduce emotional intensity, what are your top five favorites that you'd like to use for coping?

Why did you pick those five activities? Imagine yourself using them. What is most helpful about each activity?

Make a Crisis Plan

If you've completed every section of part 1, that means you explored all the steps you need to make your personal crisis plan. I hope you feel proud of the progress you've made through each of these steps. My wish for you is that you don't have any more suicidal crises in the future, but if you do, you're now more prepared to navigate them by seeking support, soothing emotional intensity, and staying safe. Next, you'll find a crisis plan summary. Please fill it out using information from the other exercises you completed in part 1 of this journal. If you find that you're still unsure how to fill something out, please reach out to a mental health professional, loved one, or call a crisis line for assistance.

MY CRISIS PLAN

Warning signs that I'm in crisis:

Reason(s) why I want to live:

People I can contact (list their names and phone numbers) for support with:

- lifting my spirits:

- sharing my feelings:

- advice on coping:

- advice on safety:

Ways to keep myself safe:

Ways to rapidly reduce intense emotional pain:

Emergency numbers and emergency room location:

Now that you have created your crisis plan, it's important to make sure you can access it at any time. Some people take a picture of it with their phone or print it out to keep in their wallet. You can do whatever works for you, but it's crucial that you can access the plan at all times in case you start experiencing suicidal thoughts and need guidance. It can also be helpful to share your crisis plan with loved ones, a mental health professional, or trusted others who can look out for warning signs and ways to help you.

*You are worthy
of safety and support
in times of trouble.*

Please note that the crisis plan you created does not have to be permanent. In fact, you should update it as often as needed so it remains as helpful as possible.

Please take some time to reflect on what it was like going through this crisis planning process. What emotions came up? How are you feeling about your plan?

Part 2

SOOTHE EMOTIONAL PAIN

Now that you established a crisis plan, let's focus on identifying the causes of your pain. Where did your suicidal thoughts come from? Does it feel like a blur? Or can you easily pinpoint the situation that prompted your first suicidal thought? Journaling can be so powerful precisely because it provides clarity about our stories, our thoughts, and our experiences. You may wonder, *Why would anyone want to see their pain more clearly?* That's a great question.

Uncover Causes and Context

Sometimes, the act of pulling the different pieces of your story together feels validating and healing. The process can deepen your understanding of the causes of your suicidal thoughts, which can point to steps to relieve them.

Now, take some time to tell the story of your suicidal thoughts and experiences. Start wherever makes sense to you.

Know that there's no wrong way to tell your story. Be tender with yourself as you write and know that this is a judgment-free space. Don't worry about spelling, grammar, or any other writing formalities—please express yourself freely. As you write, think about which problems you may have some influence on and which ones you can't control. That information will come in handy in later sections. In the next section, we'll focus on ways you can care for yourself as you explore the context surrounding your suicidal thoughts.

True Self-Care

What do you think of when you hear the phrase *self-care*? It means a lot of different things to a lot of different people. When self-care is used to talk about going to expensive spas or on fancy vacations or as a simple fix for life's stressors, I usually tune that out. Many people can't afford those luxuries as self-care, and I'm not convinced they work that well for maintaining day-to-day mental health anyway. There are stressors that become present again as soon as we step back into our lives, even after a pleasant escape.

At its core, I think of true self-care as a way to look out for yourself however you're able. This may include getting more rest or nourishment, setting healthy boundaries, practicing self-compassion, letting go of self-criticism, cultivating spiritual and other connections, limiting social media, standing up for yourself, or reserving time for fun and enjoyment. Meeting your needs may reduce your vulnerability to the type of emotional stress that prompts suicidal thoughts.

In your life, what do you have control over when it comes to taking care of yourself? What kind of self-care makes you feel you're at your best?

Please pull out the ways you tend to nourish your well-being from your writing and list them below. Take some time to set an intention to prioritize these self-care activities by writing about how you will put them into action.

Great work identifying how you can implement self-care activities in your life!

What obstacles tend to get in the way of self-care? How can you address those hurdles when you come across them? If you're not sure how, you can try out the tools in the next section focused on problem-solving.

Problem-Solve

In the previous sections, you took important steps toward soothing emotional pain by identifying causes and choosing strategies for caring for yourself as you process emotions.

Similarly, let's take time to identify some of the problems in your life and raise your awareness around them.

After you've considered the problems above, pick one that you view as having at least some control over. Then, brainstorm possible solutions for this problem.

At the brainstorming stage, all possibilities should be considered, no matter how impractical or unlikely they seem. This open, flexible approach generates multiple potential pathways to solving problems that cause emotional pain in your life.

Which solutions seem like they will be most helpful to you? Which one is the most realistic for addressing your problems?

Take some time to create action plans for how you will pursue solutions. Please make your plans specific. You will be more likely to follow through with them. If obstacles come up while you write, take some time to ponder how you could deal with them and still execute your action plans.

Amazing work—you've now zoomed out and reflected on these specific problem-solving steps to soothe sources of emotional pain:
1. Define the problem.
2. Brainstorm possible solutions.
3. Select the best solution(s) and take action.

How do you feel after processing your problems through this problem-solving framework?

How will you use this problem-solving approach when issues come up in the future? How can you remind yourself of the steps?

My deep hope is that you feel empowered and more capable of problem-solving after thinking through solutions to some of the challenges you face. This three-step problem-solving approach may seem simple, but it can really help you to move forward when you're struggling. If you feel stuck at this point, please know that it's not your fault. Life definitely includes problems that we have different levels of control over. Sometimes we have full control and other times we have zero control. Most of the time, we have at least some amount of control or influence. Those are the types of situations where the problem-solving technique is most useful. Please also consider seeking support from a therapist, loved one, mentor, clergy, or crisis line to help you figure out solutions if you still don't know what steps to take.

Analyze Painful Thoughts

When a problem can't be solved, it helps to stop and take some time to think, *How am I interpreting this problem*? Once you're aware of this, it opens the possibility of considering alternative, less painful perspectives. That may sound a bit abstract or challenging at first, but it gets easier when we break it down into smaller steps.

To begin, what is a current situation that's causing you strife? Contemplate the details through the five W framework that journalists often use to describe the main points of the subject they're reporting on: the who, what, when, where, *and* why *of the situation. Let's start with the first 4 W's in this prompt and leave the* why *for a bit later.*

I saved the *why* of the situation for last because it's most important for identifying our thoughts about situations in our lives.

Take some time to reflect on why you think this problem exists right now. Feel free to draw, write, or use a list—whatever feels most useful to capture your interpretations about the causes of your problem. In addition, what are your thoughts about how you're coping with the situation?

Our thoughts and feelings are tightly linked. For example, imagine you're at the store and you see a friend. You wave at the friend and say "Hi!" but the friend doesn't respond. If your interpretation is, *My friend's ignoring me. They must be mad at me*, you'll likely feel sad, embarrassed, or even worried about why they're angry with you.

Now, imagine your first interpretation is, *They probably didn't hear me*, or *They must be preoccupied right now*. How would you feel then? You might feel neutral or even a bit concerned about your friend.

Similarly, your thoughts and behavior influence each other. If you believe the friend didn't say hello because they're mad at you, your behavior might be to avoid them. If you think they didn't hear you or were distracted by something, your action might be to reach out later and say, "I saw you at the grocery store today, but I don't think you heard me say 'Hi.' Is everything okay?"

The triangular model of how thoughts, emotions, and behaviors influence each other is at the core of cognitive behavioral therapy (CBT).

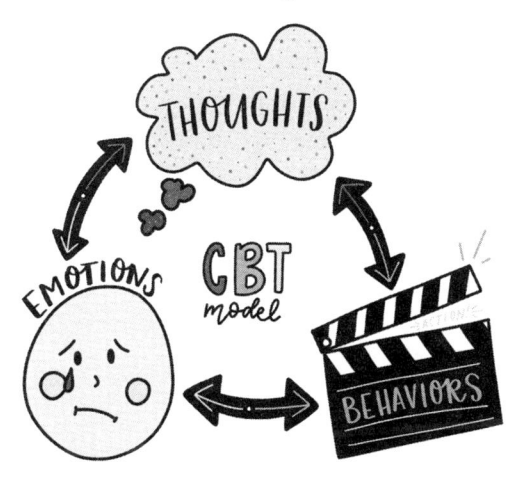

The CBT model, depicting the reciprocal relationships between thoughts, behaviors, and feelings. Illustration by Alyse Ruriani.

I remember the first time I learned about this model and understood how thoughts, emotions, and behaviors influence each other. I felt this sudden sense of clarity that my thoughts are interpretations rather than facts. This powerful awareness allowed me to shift from viewing my initial interpretations as definitive reality to first observing my thoughts and then evaluating them against evidence instead. This two-step process was particularly important for coping with the negative thoughts about myself that spurred immensely painful emotions, like shame and disgust.

Before learning about CBT, I used to think when I made a mistake, *I never do anything right.* Or if I faced a challenge, I thought, *I'll never figure this out.* Understandably, those thoughts led me to feel helpless and anticipate a gloomy future ahead. These days, I have those types of thoughts much less frequently—though I still do experience them from time to time. Our initial thoughts are often automatic and not something we can control. But now I know I can take a step back and evaluate my thoughts before feeling and acting as though they're true. I can check the evidence to see if my thoughts are realistic and useful. That gives me space to feel more capable and hopeful as I face hard times.

I'm honored to share these steps with you in the next section and hope you experience similar feelings of relief. First, I'm curious about what you're thinking and feeling after reading through this last section.

Is the CBT model already familiar to you? If so, what are your experiences with it so far? Is the CBT model sparking new insights? Are you curious, hopeful, skeptical, or experiencing another type of reaction to the CBT approach? However you feel and whatever you think, please write about it here. It's all understandable and okay.

Thank you for contemplating the CBT model. Acknowledging your painful thoughts, feelings, and actions can be hard. That's why so many of us are tempted to avoid them. But, in the long term, this awareness allows us to use coping tools that meaningfully ease the pain we're experiencing. I appreciate you approaching the rest of the CBT prompts with openness to the possibility that they may help you, even if you're unsure.

Have you ever had someone tell you that positive thinking is the way to feel better? Have you been told to just stop overthinking something? I see this on social media, in pop psychology books, and have definitely experienced it firsthand. How do you feel when someone says these types of things to you?

If you're like me and many of the patients I've treated, it feels frustrating or dismissive to be told to just change your mindset. If it were easy to *think positively*, you would already be doing it! When you're feeling suicidal, your mind has a pull toward the negative and painful. It can feel impossible to overcome that by just thinking positive thoughts.

I want to assure you that CBT is not just about thinking positively or denying the reality of your feelings—far from it. In fact, the first step of CBT is acknowledging your thoughts, feelings, and actions with warmth and curiosity. For example, you can tell yourself, *I'm learning about my thoughts, feelings, and behaviors right now. I feel compassion for myself as I explore this suffering and seek ways to soothe it.*

What are some other ways you can validate and encourage yourself as you examine your thoughts more closely?

Great job spending time thinking about how you can be gentle with yourself as you check the evidence for and against your thoughts. The good news: CBT doesn't demand that you force yourself to be optimistic to experience its benefits. Instead, CBT guides you to more accurate appraisals of yourself and the situation you're in through a series of practical steps. Through this process, you can distance yourself from the shadow that suicidal thoughts cast over you.

What do you notice about your thinking patterns when you're in a crisis or feeling suicidal? Do you unfairly criticize yourself, imagine the worst possible outcomes, or only see the bad sides of situations?

Now, let's revisit the challenging situation you journaled about earlier. What did you write for the *why* part? Rewrite your interpretation below and add the emotions that you feel and the actions it inspires alongside it. For example, you might start your sentences with the prompts below.

I interpret this situation as (identify your thoughts):

This interpretation is linked to feeling (explore the emotions):

These thoughts and feelings make me want to (reflect on the actions or behavior urges):

If you find it helpful to link your writing about thoughts, emotions, and behaviors visually, then fill in the triangular model below.

THOUGHTS:

EMOTIONS:

BEHAVIORS:

Reframe Painful Thoughts

In the next part, we'll explore ways to reframe your painful thoughts and interpretations. First, let's try getting curious about your thoughts. Reflecting on the thought(s) you identified for the situation above, are any hurtful thinking patterns present? For example:

- Are you unintentionally amplifying the negative and downplaying or ignoring the positive?
- Are you jumping to any conclusions about what the future holds or how others perceive you?
- Are you making assumptions about what someone was thinking?
- Are you thinking about the situation through an all-or-nothing lens?

What was it like exploring your thought patterns in this situation? I hope you found it helpful, leading into the deeper analysis in the next part.

Take a step back and be as objective as possible. What is the evidence leading you to believe your interpretations about the situation are true? Explore all the reasons so we can make sure we're fairly evaluating your thoughts. Try to avoid *it feels true* as an example of evidence. While your feelings are important, we know that they're impacted by the thoughts you're having. Look to see if there's additional evidence beyond your emotions that supports your interpretation as true.

For balance, let's look at the other side here. What is the evidence against your thought? Is there more context that your initial assumption was missing? Were you stating something with certainty that is actually unknown? Are there other possible outcomes? Are there other possible explanations?

If you're struggling to come up with ideas, you can try a thought exercise. Imagine you're not in the center of the situation. Instead, you're an outside person watching the situation unfold on TV or reading about it in a book. What might that observer say about the situation, and how might they interpret it?

Each step of the CBT process is important. If you skip ahead to the last step of reframing, it's hard to create a compelling reinterpretation of the situation that resonates or rings true for you. That's why we wait to come up with new interpretations until you've considered the evidence.

How are you feeling about your initial interpretations after going through this process so far? Do you view the situation any differently? If not, do you want to retry these prompts with another situation in your life that might fit better?

After working through the situation, do you have any reframed interpretations? If so, what are they? How do you feel when you have these new interpretations instead of the initial thought(s)? What emotions come up for you? Do new actions or behavior urges come up?

How are you feeling about this situation now? My hope is that it feels less painful to you—that you uncovered alternative interpretations and more context for the situation. Importantly, your participation in this process allowed you to acquire and practice a new tool. When you're feeling painful emotions, now you know you can observe the thoughts, feelings, and behaviors of the situation. Next, you can explore alternative interpretations and what the facts suggest is the most truthful, fair interpretation. Finally, you can embrace the reframed thought(s) and new emotions and the comfort they bring.

Are there future situations where you think these tools would be particularly helpful? What are they? How can you remind yourself of these coping strategies the next time you need them?

Sometimes, it's hard to believe the reframed thoughts. I've experienced this myself and have heard patients say, "I know that this is rationally true, but it doesn't *feel* true." Changing your whole way of thinking about situations, emotions, thoughts, behaviors, and how they're all connected is a lot! It's rare (maybe impossible) for everything to click into place after using CBT one time.

My suggestion is to practice this skill repeatedly until it starts to feel like second nature. It gets easier with repetition and usually starts to feel like a more natural way of thinking. You'll get the hang of this. I believe in you. As a practical suggestion, I recommend to patients that they write reframed thoughts on a piece of paper or in a note in their phones, so that they can remind themselves when their mind starts to slip into old patterns.

How can you amplify and remember your reframed thoughts when you're struggling?

What thoughts, ideas, and feelings did you have while reading and writing through this chapter? Were there certain parts you didn't relate to? Which parts felt most helpful? What did you learn? What insights did you have?

Last, I want to share a reframe I've found particularly helpful during my own mental health journey in case you find it helpful in yours. When I'm struggling to change a habit or behavior, and I repeat the unwanted behavior, I used to think, *I failed again; I'll never change.*

Instead, I now say to myself, *No wonder I'm having a hard time changing this; challenges keep coming up that interfere.* Rather than suffering the demotivating effects of viewing myself as a failure, this reframe gives me the space to identify and understand the obstacles. If I can accept myself and the persistence of the obstacles, I have a better chance of effectively navigating them the next time. Change is still possible.

Part 3

NURTURE SELF-COMPASSION

Wherever you are and however you're feeling right now, I hope you can take a moment to feel proud of working on your mental health. So often when we're struggling, we blame ourselves for not *just snapping out of it* or making quicker changes. This leads to more misery.

In this part of the journal, we'll focus on skills for relating to yourself in a compassionate manner. This is always important, but it's especially important in situations where the problem-solving and CBT strategies haven't helped to soothe the pain you're experiencing. As a reminder, this journal was designed to offer you a variety of strategies for soothing pain so you can select what works for you at any given moment.

To start, how do you generally relate to yourself? Are you compassionate and validating? Are you critical and deprecating? How do you treat yourself?

At what moments and situations do you tend to be harsher and more self-critical?

At what moments and situations do you tend to be more encouraging and kinder to yourself?

Now that you've explored how you relate to yourself, where do you think this pattern comes from? Is the way you treat yourself influenced by past or current relationships? Did certain situations or circumstances evoke this pattern? Have you always related to yourself this way, or did it change at some point?

Take some time to explore and understand how you got to this point. Be soft with yourself as you process these experiences, as I imagine some may be quite painful.

Experiences of Discrimination

We live in a world with inequities, and tragically, that means people who hold marginalized identities may face more stressors and oppression than other people. If you hold any marginalized identities related to your race, ethnicity, sexual orientation, gender identity, abilities, religion, age, financial situation, appearance, or other characteristics, the discrimination in your life may increase the risk for suicidal thoughts. This may have affected you in systemic (for instance, difficulty accessing housing, medical care, education, and employment) and individual matters (for instance, bullying, harassment, and violence).

It's heartbreaking that people who hold marginalized identities may unintentionally internalize societal biases and blame themselves for the discrimination they face. This may be especially true if you're surrounded by people who hold prejudices toward you or think that discrimination is a thing of the past.

I'd like you to take some time to reflect on how societal biases affect how you view yourself and your experiences. This is a safe, private space for you to write.

Please be gentle with yourself as you explore these questions and memories. My sincere hope is that by journaling about them, together we can find a way for you to reject societal messages that undermine your self-worth. No aspect of your identity diminishes your right to a radiant life.

Please remember to stop any time you feel like the exercise is leading to more intense suicidal thoughts and contact a crisis line if you need to talk to someone right away. Please skip any sections that don't serve you or that don't apply to you.

Have you ever experienced discrimination, prejudice, or mistreatment that's linked to your suicidal thoughts? For example, have you been bullied, teased, or excluded from jobs, housing, education, or healthcare because of an identity you hold?

Have those experiences contributed to a negative view of yourself? How so?

How have these experiences influenced your suicidal thoughts? Do you remember certain incidents that prompted suicidal thoughts? Who did you turn to for support? How did you try to take care of yourself when this happened?

I'm so sorry that you experienced the injustice of bias and discrimination. I'm confident that you truly belong in this world. You're worthy of all of the good parts of life. The inequities of the world aren't your fault. I hope you can take these messages to heart. The world can be hard enough without you blaming yourself for these painful experiences.

What would it look like to be an ally for yourself? How can you validate yourself and your feelings even after you've had invalidating or discriminatory experiences?

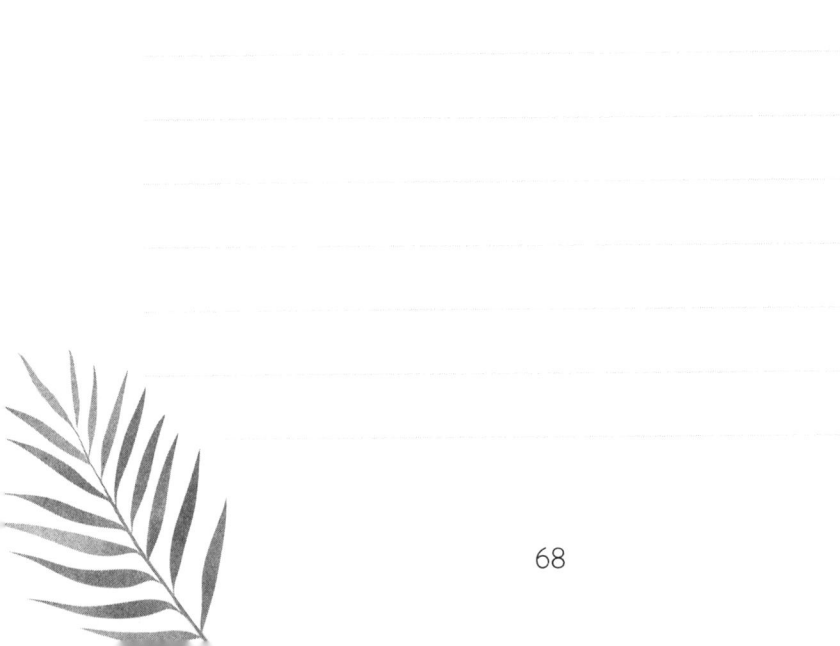

Self-Validation

If you get sick with the flu, a cold, or a sore throat, how do you respond to that? I hope that you find time to rest, drink plenty of fluids, and allow yourself time to heal. Is your approach to medical illness different from your approach to your emotional well-being and mental health? How are they similar or different? If they're discrepant, why is that?

I asked you to contemplate differences between tending to mental and physical health because I hope to show you that, in times of vulnerability, you need extra self-care and compassion. I hope that if you show yourself some kindness when you're medically ill, you're able to carry those behaviors over to times you're feeling emotionally unwell or facing stressors. What would it be like to tell yourself statements like, *I'm going through something upsetting, My frustration and hurt are valid,* or *I deserve extra tenderness as I work through this*?

If that would be hard for you, what gets in the way of relating to yourself with compassion? Do you think you don't deserve it? If so, is there someone in your life who has supported and validated you in the past? How would they respond to you when you're in pain? What would it take to channel that response toward yourself?

After reflecting on what you've written for this section, what types of situations do you think self-validation would be helpful for in the future?

Your Sources of Strength

Are there cultural values, traditions, or communities related to your identity that have served as sources of strength? For example, some people find pride and support from spiritual communities, LGBTQIA2S+ organizations, cultural centers, or family traditions. What communities give you a sense of strength and connection?

If you couldn't think of any communities that give you strength, would you be open to seeking some out? Whether in person or online, what kinds of communities could you reach out to for strength? Where would you like to explore? Please keep in mind that communities can be related to some part of your identity, but they can also be related to common interests (for instance, reading, playing games, photography, listening to or playing music, martial arts, cooking, politics, or sports).

Write about how you can act on finding communities that serve as sources of strength.

Finally, I'd like you to think about other sources you can turn to for strength. Are there pieces of art, quotes, or certain places that you can look to for reminders of your worth?

If you're having a hard time finding resources, please see the crisis numbers at the beginning of this journal. Please know that you can reach out to those resources to ask for help with finding communities that suit your needs. Public libraries can also be an excellent resource for connecting you with literature and media that are relevant to you.

What Would You Tell a Friend?

This section focuses on more ways to cultivate self-compassion. Sometimes, it's so hard for us to show ourselves compassion even though we show it to others in our lives. Think about a stressful situation you went through recently where you responded to yourself with blame and criticism. Reflect on the details of the situation, including how you felt when you were mean to yourself.

Now, I want you to imagine that the situation happened to your friend instead of yourself. What would you say to your friend? How would you comfort them?

What was it like trying the what would I tell a friend strategy? *Did you respond to your friend differently than you responded to yourself? If not, how come? If you did, why do you think that is?*

What do you need to get a place where you can be friendly to yourself? Set a plan to encourage and comfort yourself in future times of distress. What does that look like? What are some ways you can practice greeting yourself with compassion?

Show Yourself Kindness

I went out to get coffee while I was writing this book. When the barista handed me the cup, it had two stickers: a flower and a message saying, *Be kind to yourself today.* I'm not proud to say my first instinct was to roll my eyes (yes, I see the irony!). I realized it felt vulnerable to be kind to myself instead of pushing myself in various ways. Taking a deep breath, I looked at the message again and viewed it as a sweet reminder instead of an irritation.

I share this because we all face obstacles to fully embracing these coping strategies—even those of us who've been practicing them for years, like me. That doesn't mean we're failing. It means that we can keep working on new ways of relating to ourselves and giving ourselves grace, even when our initial reactions push against them.

With that in mind, have you ever had someone close to you struggle with suicidal thoughts? If so, how did you express your support? If you haven't known anyone else who struggles with suicidal thoughts, what would you do for a loved one who started to struggle?

Hopefully, that last reflection opened you up to thinking about what you need when you're suffering. It's important to acknowledge that different people need different things when they're suffering.

What do you need when you're having suicidal thoughts?

After reflecting on how you would show up for others and what you need, what are some ways you can show yourself kindness? Are there certain affirmations you can say to yourself? Are there certain people you can reach out to or favorite places you can go to? Are there activities you can do that feel good?

What gets in the way of you showing up for yourself in a kind way when you struggle? What can you do to overcome those hurdles in the future?

Cultivate Acceptance

Now that we've spent some time with self-compassion, let's pivot to a related concept: acceptance. In this specific context, acceptance isn't about approving of reality. It's about acknowledging reality as it is right now. Many therapeutic, religious, and philosophical approaches include a focus on acceptance as a pathway to peace. This reveals that it's a common human inclination to push away painful and frustrating parts of reality, and that suffering tends to lessen when you accept reality.

One example where this was at play is when the COVID-19 pandemic began in 2020. Our lives turned upside down as we faced enormous changes. Suddenly, seemingly mundane daily activities like school, work, getting groceries, and seeing friends completely transformed. This all happened against a heartbreaking backdrop of many people becoming ill and losing their lives. Many of us struggled to accept that reality and wanted to deny that it was happening. It was too painful to fully believe.

Yet, in those painful times, hope also emerged when people acknowledged reality. People figured out creative and safe ways to connect, to engage with hobbies, to cope, and to reduce the risk of COVID-19 exposure. Although we wished that the new pandemic reality wasn't true, we knew there was nothing we could do to change it. Accepting reality allowed us to hold compassion for ourselves and each other in a painful time. It gave us space to find ways to cope the best we could. That's the power of acknowledgment. It doesn't fix the situation, but it allows us to feel less stuck in denial. It allows us to move forward and stop fighting truths we can't change.

Thinking back on the situations you've endured in your life—personal or as part of a larger community—what's your relationship with acceptance? Have you found it useful in your life? What do you view as benefits of accepting reality?

What insights did you have as you wrote? One of the major benefits of accepting reality is that it allows you to acknowledge the true situation, see what's needed, and then choose your next steps. The more painful the reality, the harder it can be to do this.

Let's take some time to contemplate approaches to cultivating acceptance. What's a situation in your life right now that would be helpful for you to accept? Remember that acceptance can only focus on the past or present because we don't know the future yet. Is the situation about yourself, someone else, or a situation happening in the world? Are you focused on a regret or current situation? Please include the details as you write.

What would it look like to accept this situation? What steps could you take to help you to accept the situation? What would the benefits be?

If you can't accept this situation right now, that's okay. This is the type of skill that requires continued work. Sometimes, the focus is on accepting yourself and your feelings as they are—with kindness and compassion—rather than feeling shame or getting frustrated with yourself. If this is where your head's at right now, try to find a comfortable space and just imagine what it would be like to accept yourself and your feelings as they are right now. What can you say to encourage yourself as you picture this? If you're struggling to find words, here are a few examples I hope you'll find helpful.

- *My situation is painful right now. It's understandable that acceptance is hard for me.*
- *I acknowledge the reality that I struggle with acceptance. I'm proud of myself for staying open to finding new ways to try to accept painful situations.*
- *At this moment, I accept every part of my feelings, including my desire to reject reality.*

What would you add to the statements above? Do you find it helpful to pray (for instance, the "Serenity Prayer"), meditate, read (for example, Virginia Satir's poem, "My Declaration of Self-Esteem"), or listen to certain songs (for instance, "Let It Be")?

Select some sources of inspiration for acceptance and write about how you'll use them to cultivate acceptance.

Write a supportive letter to yourself about the challenges you currently face. With warmth, ask yourself to consider accepting areas of your life and yourself that you would like to accept but are having trouble with right now.

I hope writing a letter to yourself provided the embrace and nurturing you need as you continue to work on yourself and your mental health. *How are you feeling after writing about self-compassion and acceptance?* I hope that these practices lead you to less self-blame, less denial, and less shame about your feelings. *Finally, what kind of situations can you apply these self-compassion and acceptance tools to in the future?*

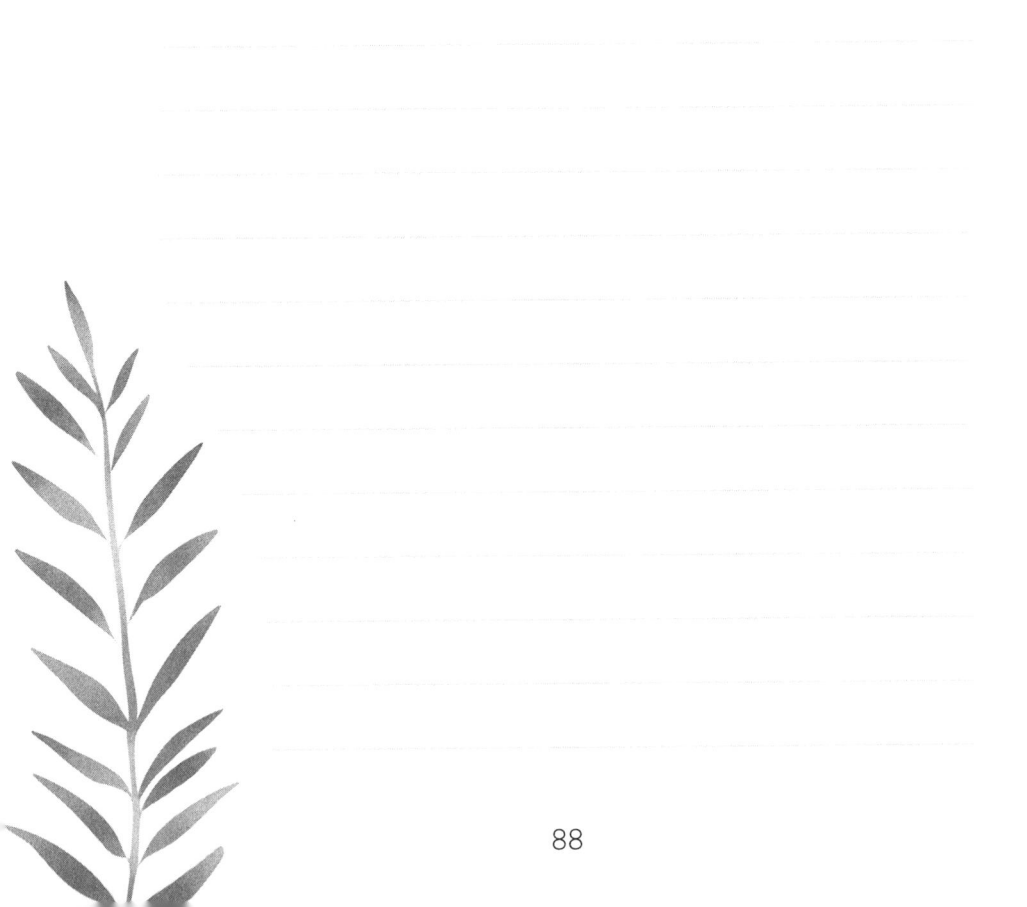

Part 4

BUILD HOPE

When you experience suicidal thoughts, it can feel like you'll never be okay again. You might fear a life that's devoid of joy forever. In these excruciating moments, the belief in a possibility for better days can keep you holding on. Sadly, it can be the hardest to find hope when you need it the most. In part 4, we'll look at ways to find hope together so you have support and strategies to help you through your struggles.

Let's start by exploring your experiences with hope. Which parts of your life lead you to feel hopeless in this present moment? What does that feel like for you? What kinds of thoughts, feelings, physical sensations, and behaviors do you have when you're in this state?

Now, let's look at the flip side; when you're in immense pain, where do you turn for glimmers of hope? What keeps you holding on? What are your main reasons for pushing through another day?

How do you feel after reflecting on the reasons you feel hopeless and hopeful?

When suicidal thoughts take over your mind, the world is overshadowed by suffering. This isn't your fault. It's a particularly challenging part of the way mental health works. Your mind more easily finds reasons to reinforce your sense of despair than reasons to counteract them. In that headspace, it's hard to find sparks of light, illuminating sources of hope.

I created tools explicitly for guiding you to find hope during the hardest moments. They are captured in the HOPE acronym:

- (seek) Help
- (find) Optimism
- (change) Perspective
- (attend to) Emotions.

Please keep in mind that these aren't intended to be four sequential steps you must follow to find hope. Instead, they're a menu of options for finding hope. You can select whichever works best for you in any given moment, matching your energy and capability level.

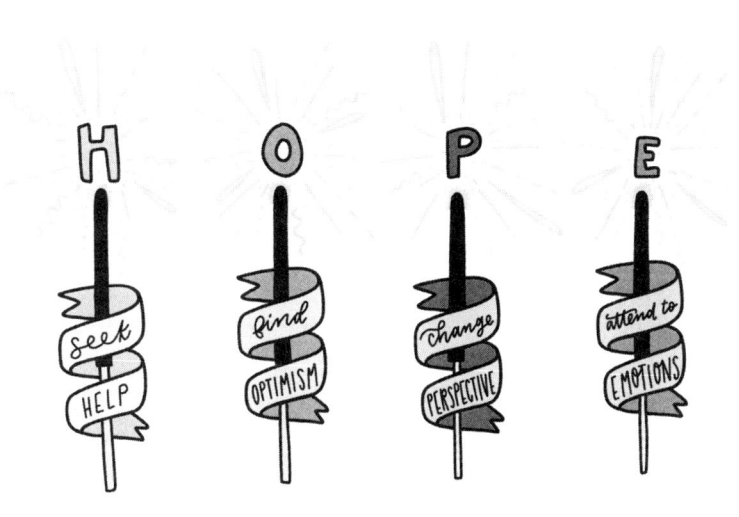

Four approaches to building hope: seeking help, finding optimism, changing perspective, and attending to emotions. Illustration by Alyse Ruriani.

Seek Help

When you're feeling hopeless, who helps you find hope? Are there special people in your life that help you believe in the possibility of a better future? Do you have people who bring you joy despite all that feels wrong right now? Who are those people?

They can be friends, family, coworkers, mental health professionals, peer supports—whoever comes to mind. Picture them and identify what it is about them that helps you experience hope.

If you can't think of anyone, please think about people you could potentially seek help from next time you feel hopeless. What is the name of a person or organization you can seek help from? How and when will you contact them? What kind of help will you ask for?

The more specific you are, the more likely you'll be to follow through with your intention of seeking help. If you don't know where to start, consider calling one of the crisis lines at the beginning of this book for referrals and suggestions.

What obstacles stand in the way of you seeking help from others? Do you feel unworthy? Do you feel like you should do it all on your own? Are you unsure about how to ask for what you need? Reflect on those obstacles and ways to overcome them.

Strategies might include writing out what you want to say when you ask for help, reminding yourself that seeking help is a sign of strength, and remembering that you're worthy of assistance. We all need help at some point or another in our lives.

How did your reflections on help-seeking go? If you found yourself thinking, *No one gives me hope or can give me hope*, please don't give up. We can expand our options.

Are there people you don't personally know that help you to feel hopeful? Is there an artist, musician, athlete, community leader, comedian, mentor, or other person who has made it through struggles you relate to? Do you feel hope from their stories? Who are they? Include pictures, lyrics, quotes, or whatever it is that reminds you of them so you can reach for it when you're in need of a boost.

If you're still feeling unsure, that's okay. Let's brainstorm about other people you can draw support from when you're having a hard time finding hope.

Are there fictional characters from books, movies, comic books, plays, or elsewhere that inspire you? Who are they? How can you make the hope they inspire more memorable to you? Are there places you can keep their picture, quotes, or other bits of wisdom?

Find Optimism

When you're feeling suicidal, your perspective can become so clouded that you only see the worst parts of the world. The good news is that you can break through those clouds when you find real reasons for optimism. Let's start by exploring what you have to look forward to.

Is there anything, big or small, that you're excited about? Are there things you would be sad to miss out on if you weren't here anymore? As you contemplate these, please be specific (for instance, sunsets, breezy days, being with family, seeing a child grow up, having coffee or tea in the morning, a sequel to a movie you really want to see, or following your favorite sports team).

You can also uncover reasons for optimism by examining evidence from past experiences. What hardships have you been able to get through that you initially viewed as insurmountable?

When we get past troubled times, it's human nature to just move on. Life can be so busy that it's hard to truly reflect and give yourself credit for what you've survived. Or we may not want to think about the bad times once we're through them because it's hard to look back. Bringing those experiences to mind can remind us that we can get through our current difficulties too.

Let's take a deeper dive. How did you get through that challenge? Explore the strengths, skills, and resources you used to get through that situation.

In light of the evidence you just explored, what helps you to feel more confident about your current challenges? How can you use the resources you used in past situations in your current situation? Allow this to build your confidence for facing current and future challenges.

May that past evidence light the path for hope through the current challenges you face.

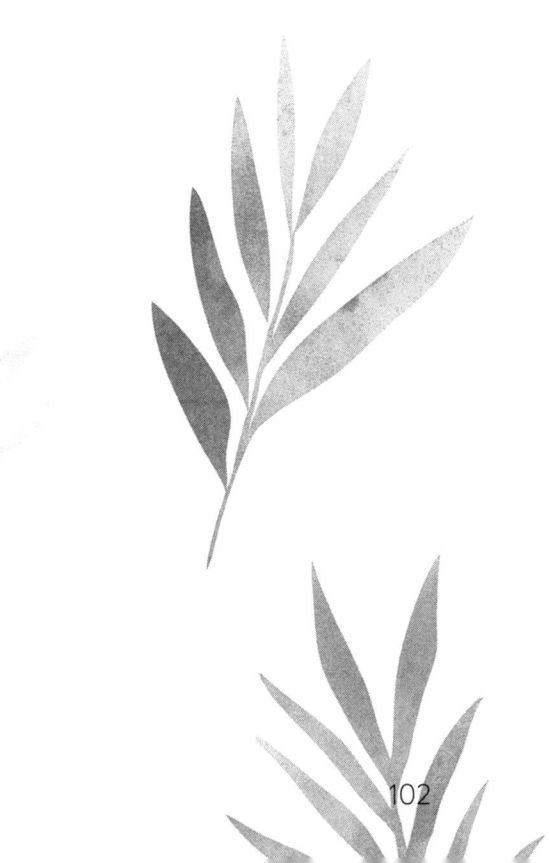

Change Perspective

Why do some folks feel hopeless when others seem effortlessly hopeful? The reasons are complex and include life circumstances, fortune, societal privilege, and how much support is available to buffer against stress. In addition, an important factor related to hope is how we interpret the causes and outcomes of stressful situations.

Imagine you get into a car accident. Many different pieces will factor into your level of hopelessness, including the extent of the damage, how badly you or other passengers were hurt, and the implications you see for the future. In addition, your interpretation of the cause and the outcome of the car accident will influence your level of hopelessness. Specifically, if you view it as 100% your fault (internal attribution), related to you as a whole (global), and unchanging or forever bad (stable), intense hopelessness will arise.

Meanwhile, if you view the accident as something the other driver or the weather played a part in (contribution of external forces), an unfortunate accident without implications for other areas of yourself or your life (specific), and something that isn't part of a string of endless tragic events in your life (unstable), you won't feel hopeless.

Of course, you're not intentionally trying to view situations negatively. Stressful situations impact us differently depending on what they mean to us. Once you're aware of these patterns, you can find new perspectives for situations with CBT approaches. Remember that CBT isn't about trying to just look at the positive or lie to yourself so you feel better. It's about seeking out evidence you may have missed in your initial interpretation. This enables you to generate more realistic, helpful beliefs.

Think about a current stressful situation you're in. Do you blame yourself for it and if so, why?

Are there any external factors that were not in your control? What are they? Even if it's your fault, can you give yourself some grace? Were you doing the best you knew how to at the time? Would you equally blame a friend in the same situation as you? If not, why? Reflect on ways to shift your perspective from total internal blame to consider the broader context and other external factors.

Global interpretations of situations include beliefs like, *This situation means something about my overall worth as a person.*

Does this apply to how you're thinking about your current situation? If so, let's think about some other possible perspectives. Have you been in a similar situation to this one with a better outcome? Are you unintentionally overly focused on negative experiences and ignoring positive ones? What areas of your life will not be affected by this situation? Are there actions you can take to minimize the spread of the negative impact in your life?

How are you feeling after your reflection above? Were you able to shift your thoughts to something more specific to the situation instead of something global about who you are and your life as a whole? What are your current interpretations of the situation?

Stable interpretations include thoughts such as, *Nothing will ever get better.* Understandably, this belief really turns the volume up on feelings of defeat.

Can you identify past challenging situations where things unexpectedly turned out well? Are there ways to influence the situation to create a better outcome? If you and the situation truly won't change, is it possible the way you feel about it could change? Are there people in similar situations with different outlooks that inspire you?

After pondering the questions in the last section, do you view your situation differently? If you're feeling more hopeful, what led to the change?

Attend to Emotions

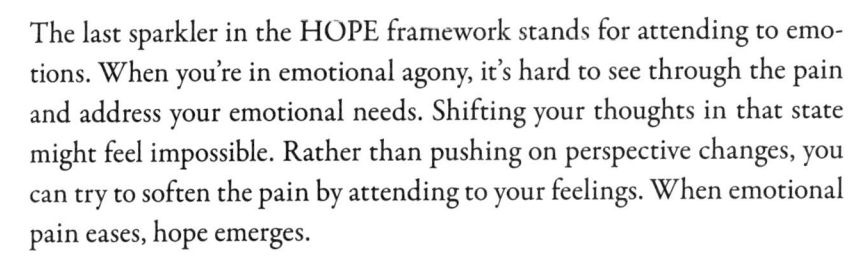

The last sparkler in the HOPE framework stands for attending to emotions. When you're in emotional agony, it's hard to see through the pain and address your emotional needs. Shifting your thoughts in that state might feel impossible. Rather than pushing on perspective changes, you can try to soften the pain by attending to your feelings. When emotional pain eases, hope emerges.

To start, focus on how you're feeling right now. What prompted your current emotions? If you're not sure, that's okay. If you want to focus on a past situation where you experienced different emotions for this part of writing, that's okay too. Please pick the situation that works best for you.

Now, take a moment to validate your feelings and thank yourself for focusing on your well-being, even when it's hard. What do you think your current emotions are communicating to you? What do you need?

What action(s) can you take to soothe your painful emotions? How can you get your needs met? If you're feeling stuck in this area, keep in mind that it's often a trial-and-error process to find what you need. The important part is that you keep trying and give yourself credit for your efforts.

Have you ever read a sad news story or listened to a sad song and noticed that it makes your thoughts about the world overall feel grimmer? Maybe you think more negative thoughts like, *The world is full of despair.* That's because your emotions and thoughts influence each other, as you'll recall from the CBT model. Awareness of these reciprocal relationships gives you the power to influence them. Specifically, you can try to alleviate grim thoughts by seeking emotional levity.

What soothes hurtful emotions? What lifts you up? Explore what has worked for you in the past and why you find it helpful.

What are some uplifts you'd like to try next time you're feeling hopeless? If you're not sure, remember that these can be simple (for example, listening to a song you love, watching a favorite movie, drinking a cup of tea, coloring, playing a game, taking a hot shower, or snuggling your favorite person or pet) or more involved (for example, listening to live music, taking a scenic walk or drive, baking or cooking a meal you enjoy, or creating a poem or piece of art).

Get curious and creative to discover what works best for you. This is an opportunity to be flexible and explore. If you find something has a negative effect on you in any way, discard it and try another option.

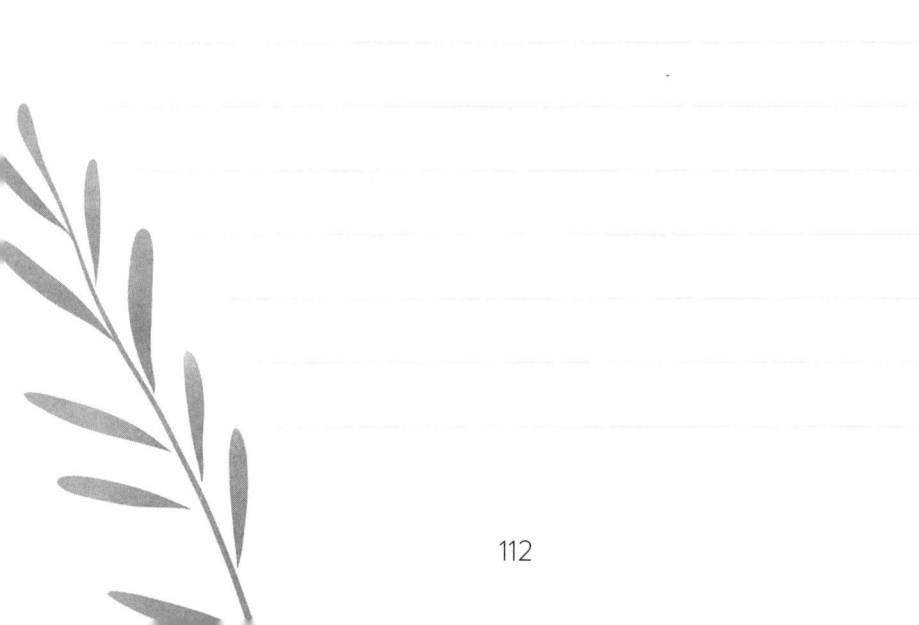

When you're in a low or painful mood, it can be hard to come up with ways to feel better. I suggested creating an easily accessible running list of things to try that you can update with your favorite activities. Sometimes, just knowing you have some options is an empowering experience in and of itself. Remember, if you don't feel completely better from these actions, that's okay and normal. The goal is to try to lift your mood and level of hope bit by bit.

Emotional pain can blunt the effects of joyful and pleasant activities. That's why you may feel like there's no point in engaging in them when you feel down. If you view emotional uplifts as ways to increase joy and pleasure alongside (instead of replacing) the pain, your motivation to try the activities may increase. Any experience of uplift, even if momentary, is evidence that the future might feel better.

How can you encourage yourself to try uplifts?

What kind of future situations will you use the tool of uplifts for? How can you see them counteracting the belief that pain is never-ending? How can they bring you hope?

Make a Hope Box

When you boil it down to its basics, hope is openness to the possibility that there may be better times ahead. It's hard to remember your reasons for living, coping skills, and other prompts for finding hope when you're feeling hopeless. One way to compile the different strategies you've uncovered in this part of the journal is to collect them in a Hope Box (sometimes called a Survival Kit; Bryan and Rudd 2018; Wenzel, Brown, and Beck 2009). Hope Boxes can include reminders of your reasons for living (like pictures or lists), goals, go-to coping strategies, your crisis plan from part 1, symbols and sentimental items that lift your spirits, or even this journal. You can design and plan your Hope Box here and then create something physical or use a digital folder on your computer or phone. You may also want to try out the free Virtual Hope Box app (Bush et al. 2015; Denneson et al. 2019).

What will you put into your Hope Box?

As you think of each item, reflect on how that may increase your sense of hope in times of need. Use as many details as you can while you plan your Hope Box and reflect on the function of each item you choose. Remember that, just like your crisis plan, a Hope Box can transform as you find new pieces to add or want to remove parts that are no longer relevant.

In this part of the journal, you learned the four components of the HOPE **frame**work and how to assemble a Hope Box. I hope these tools are useful to you.

You are worthy of hope and the light it brings.

Part 5

CONNECT WITH PEOPLE

Strengthen Connections

No journal focused on suicidal thoughts would be complete without spending time on the importance of nurturing relationships for the benefit of our physical and emotional well-being (Holt-Lunstad et al. 2015). So let's turn to that now. Anecdotally, I've seen an increase in the number of social media posts joking about not being a people person. For example, do you relate to the meme of David from *Schitt's Creek*, season 1 when he says, "I'm trying very hard not to connect with people right now"? We'll reflect on those types of urges to withdraw from people when we struggle and why it's good for our mental health to do what David ultimately does in later *Schitt's Creek* seasons: strengthen connections with friends and family.

What's your first thought at the suggestion of increasing the number of interpersonal connections you have for your well-being?

Now, let's explore what your current relationships are like. How do you feel about the people you're connected to in your life right now? Do you feel you have the amount and kind of connections you want? How often do you feel lonely?

Thank you for reflecting on your current connections. If you're happy with them, what are you doing that is working well? What do you like?

If you feel disappointed in your current relationships, please know you're not alone. Many of us find it challenging to have as many friends as we would like or to form the close connections we desire.

What steps do you think you can take to feel less lonely? Are there community activities, online groups, or hobbies you've been meaning to try that could lead to new connections? One resource I've personally found helpful is checking out the local public library, which often has a variety of free activities people can participate in, including games, arts, crafts, book clubs, guest speakers, and more. If that doesn't feel like a good fit, where else might you look for connection?

Great work brainstorming about places you could go to meet new people!

What about the current people in your life? Is there anyone you would like to get to know better or to talk to more frequently? Take some time to think about actions you would be willing to try, even if they feel a little anxiety provoking at first. Hopefully, they will lead to stronger connections and chip away at your loneliness.

You are worthy of friendship and a support network.

Explore Emotional Safety

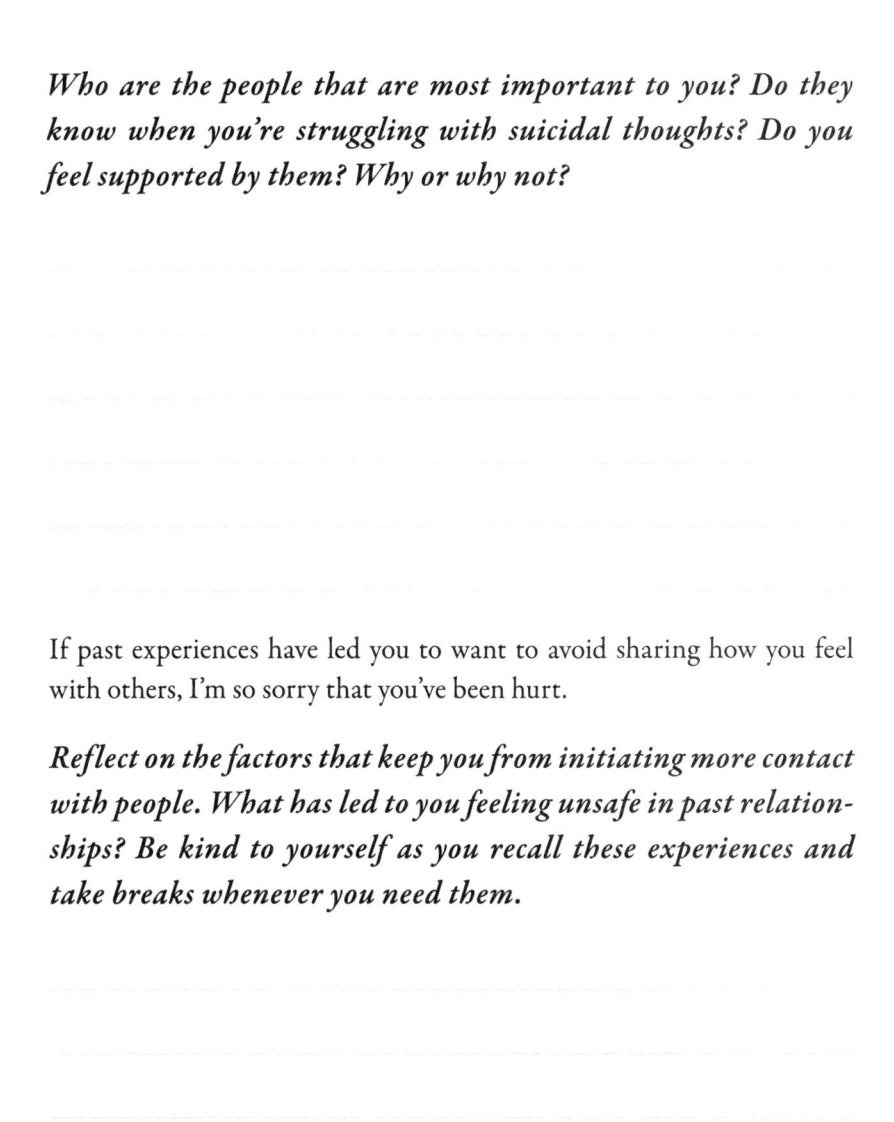

Who are the people that are most important to you? Do they know when you're struggling with suicidal thoughts? Do you feel supported by them? Why or why not?

If past experiences have led you to want to avoid sharing how you feel with others, I'm so sorry that you've been hurt.

Reflect on the factors that keep you from initiating more contact with people. What has led to you feeling unsafe in past relationships? Be kind to yourself as you recall these experiences and take breaks whenever you need them.

How do you feel writing about those memories? I want to be clear: whoever you are and whatever your past looks like, you're worthy of healthy support and connections. I respect the courage you have in reflecting on your past relationships. All relationships are definitely not created equal. As you think about building connections, let's prioritize your emotional safety by identifying what you need when you're feeling vulnerable.

Bring to mind someone you feel comfortable talking to about your feelings. Who are they? How do you feel in their presence? What is it that they do or don't do that makes you feel safe?

If you feel comfortable, consider sharing what makes you feel emotionally safe with people in your life so they can better understand how to hold a space for you when you struggle. Write, draw, or otherwise express what makes you feel most emotionally safe.

You Belong

We all have a shared need to belong (Joiner 2005; Van Orden et al. 2010). Right now, do you feel like you belong? What moments stand out in your life as a time when you felt deep belonging? If you don't feel like you belong currently, when have you felt like you belonged?

*Are there parts of your identity that have led you to feel like it's **harder** to connect? Do you feel like others judge you because of these qualities?*

If so, I'm so sorry you've experienced this. Please be kind to yourself as **you** contemplate these questions.

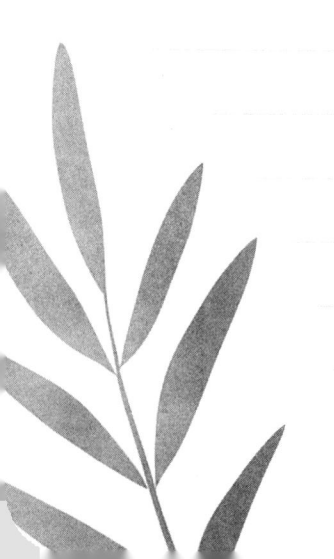

What about the other side? Are there parts of who you are that lead you to feel connected to other people and like you're part of a group? What are these groups and who are the people who help you feel like you belong? Is there a higher power or belief system you feel connected to or a spirituality that helps you feel like you belong? Are there places you can go to that feel like home to you—like a place you're meant to be? How often are you connecting with these groups and parts of yourself currently?

When you feel alone, how can you strengthen your sense of belonging? Are there parts of your identity you would like to reacquaint yourself with? Reflect and form intentions to strengthen those feelings of connection and belonging within yourself and with others.

What obstacles might get in the way on your journey to strengthen connections? How can you problem-solve around those obstacles?

Revisit "Problem-Solve" in part 2 if you're feeling unsure of the next steps. Remember that efforts to strengthen your sense of belonging don't have to be grand gestures. You can plant seeds of connection that ultimately grow into stronger relationships and fulfill your need to belong.

Above all, I want to reassure you of a key point: *you belong* in this world. I don't know you or your life situations personally, but I know that. Your experiences and the hard parts of the world may have led you to the space you're in. Please embrace yourself with love. Allow yourself to reject the forces that say you don't belong. Pay attention to people who welcome you, who believe you belong in this world. You do.

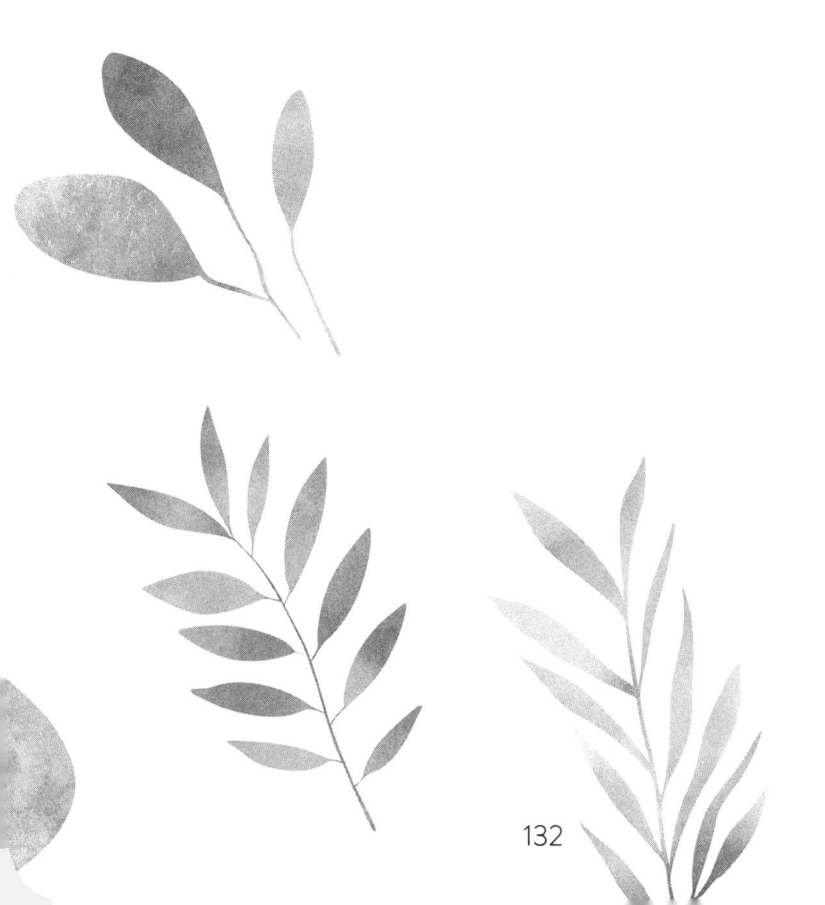

You Are Not a Burden

Tragically, many people who struggle with suicidal thoughts feel like they're a burden (Joiner 2005; Van Orden et al. 2010). Have you ever felt that way? Do you currently feel that way? Be patient with yourself as you explore this topic.

If you feel like a burden, it must ache so much. I want you to know that the people in your life wouldn't be better off without you.

Using your CBT tools, what's some evidence against your thoughts that you're a burden? Are you discounting when people say they want you in their lives? Are you downplaying your contributions to the world?

If so, spend some time reframing your thoughts in light of the evidence that you're not a burden. You can ask a trusted person for help if you're struggling to see how you make the world better and what you bring to this world.

Sometimes when you feel like a burden, gathering evidence that you aren't isn't enough to shift your beliefs. During a suicidal crisis, it can be hard to challenge thoughts, and behaviors have more of an impact.

Thinking back to the CBT model, are there behaviors you can adopt and actions you can take that reduce that sense of being a burden? Are there ways you can contribute (even a small kindness) or people you can be around that ease that feeling of being a burden? What are those actions and who are the people you can prioritize to diminish that pain? Remember to savor the positive feelings as you contribute so they chip away at the belief that you're a burden.

I'm so happy you're here and open to the possibility that you're worthy of feeling better. I hope you feel proud of all you're doing to heal.

After reflecting throughout this chapter on your current connections, feelings of belonging, and the potential of feeling like a burden, how are you doing right now? What was that like for you? If there are obstacles getting in the way of using the tools in this part of the journal, what are they? How might you work through them? Can you find ways to keep encouraging yourself?

Part 6

MAKE MEANING

In *Man's Search for Meaning,* Holocaust survivor and psychiatrist Viktor Frankl wrote about surviving concentration camps and the insights borne of his experiences (1959/2006). Frankl faced what seemed like impossible pain and hopelessness. He lost loved ones, suffered through horrible circumstances, and lived in constant fear. One of the powerful forces that kept him going was his sense of meaning. Frankl proposed that there are multiple pathways to meaning. I'm going to share them with you here so you can explore tools for building meaning in your own life.

Before we start, what do you find most meaningful in your life? Is meaning something you struggle to experience? What has that been like for you? Are there other times in your life where you've felt more meaning? What has changed? What do you think could bring more meaning to your life?

Identify Your Values

Values are whatever you wish to hold as priorities in your life. Examples may include courage, charity, justice, honesty, education, originality, passion, and many others. Our values are often connected to our sense of meaning.

What are your values? What values do you respect in others? What do you think led you to embrace these values?

Now that you've identified your values, we can dive deeper into the pathways to meaning that Frankl proposed:

- actions and experiences
- relationships
- attitudes toward unavoidable suffering.

Find Meaning in Actions and Experiences

What are some recent actions you took that align with your values? How do you feel when you participate in actions and experiences that are consistent with your values? Are there additional actions you can take that help you embrace your values? Specify what they are and reflect on a plan to carry them out. What obstacles come up for you? Explore and brainstorm ways to overcome those obstacles.

Frankl also wrote about making meaning through experiences such as goodness, truth, and beauty through nature, cultural activities, or the love of another person.

Did reading that prompt any memories of feeling awe, joy, or a strong sense of meaning? What about situations where you gained a greater perspective? Recall those experiences and how they enhance your sense of meaning.

How can you recreate those meaningful experiences? Can you pursue new ones to amplify your sense of meaning? They may involve traveling, connecting with a group that shares your interests, or even setting intentions to spend more time in places, with people, or with interests you enjoy. What hurdles might get in the way and how can you overcome them?

Find Meaning in Relationships

Which relationships mean the most in your life? When suicidal thoughts consume you, is there a person, people, or pet that pops into your mind and gives you pause about ending your life? What is it about that relationship that means so much to you?

When you struggle, you may feel like isolating yourself, even from those who mean the absolute most to you. What can you do to stay connected to meaningful relationships during times of strife?

This might look like dedicating time to reflect on the relationship, sharing your feelings with them, or making plans with them. Setting specific goals helps to execute action plans. As always, try to be realistic and recognize that seemingly small steps can have big impacts as you think about ways to connect with meaningful relationships.

Find Meaning in Suffering

Frankl also conveyed the possibility of finding meaning in suffering. Importantly, he stated he didn't believe you have to suffer to find meaning. However, if you face unavoidable suffering, it's possible to find meaning within it.

What types of suffering have you experienced in your life? What made the suffering unavoidable? Did you find any meaning from that experience? If not, that's okay. You can focus on the other paths to meaning that appear earlier in this section of the journal. Please take some time to write about your experiences of suffering to see if any sense of meaning arises as you reflect.

I'm so sorry you've experienced this type of suffering.

What was the experience like as you wrote about it? Did any themes of meaning come out of it—maybe some unanticipated insights? Did you have any changes in life priorities? Did any of your relationships change in positive ways? Did you learn anything from it?

If not, that's okay. Please focus on the other components of meaning making and be extra kind to yourself in the face of suffering. Not all suffering brings meaning, though that may evolve with time.

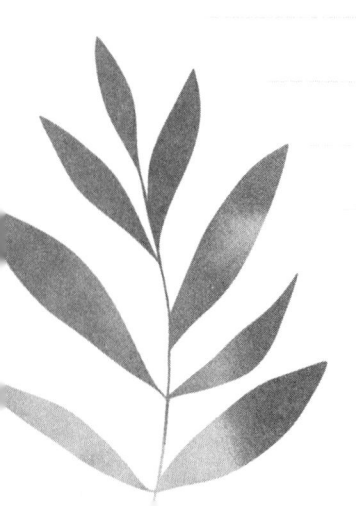

Make a Meaning Collage

Now that you've considered meaning in your life, you may find it helpful to pull all of the most important themes together in one place for you to reference whenever you need a boost. You might even consider sharing it with trusted others so they can understand you on a deeper level.

You can write more in the space below or choose to draw how you're feeling. Another option is to make a collage by collecting pictures that represent meaning and combining them here or in a separate space.

Conclusion

Wow—you made it to the last section of the guided journal. I hope you feel accomplished and have some new insights, go-to strategies, and ideas for coping with your suicidal thoughts. Your mental health is important, and I'm grateful that you've prioritized it through this process. Please take a moment to reflect on the courage you showed by taking this journey.

Looking back, what was hardest for you? How were you able to keep going during those painful parts?

As you worked through the journal, what sections have proven most helpful in your life? What had the biggest impact?

How can you continue to use your new tools and journaling practice in the future?

Overall, how has journaling made a difference in your life? What future situations do you think journaling would be helpful for?

From the bottom of my heart, thank you for the time and effort you put into this journal. It represents the best tools and insights I've come across through decades as a suicide prevention researcher, educator, and therapist. I hope you found them helpful in your life. I'm thankful you kept an open mind and gave yourself opportunities to learn new ways to navigate challenges. Whatever lies ahead, I'm wishing for the absolute best for you.

May you experience empowerment, many sparks of hope, self-compassion, and a life with deeply felt connections and meaning.

ADDITIONAL RESOURCES

Self-Help Books

Freedenthal, S. 2023. *Loving Someone with Suicidal Thoughts: What Family, Friends, and Partners Can Say and Do.* Oakland, CA: New Harbinger Publications.

Gillihan, S. J. 2022. *Mindful Cognitive Behavioral Therapy: A Simple Path to Healing, Hope, and Peace.* San Francisco: HarperOne.

Gordon, K. H. 2021. *The Suicidal Thoughts Workbook: CBT Skills to Reduce Emotional Pain, Increase Hope, and Prevent Suicide.* Oakland, CA: New Harbinger Publications.

Minden, J. 2020. *Show Your Anxiety Who's Boss: A Three-Step CBT Program to Help You Reduce Anxious Thoughts and Worry.* Oakland, CA: New Harbinger Publications.

Pettit, J. W., and R. M. Hill. 2022. *Overcoming Suicidal Thoughts for Teens: CBT Activities to Reduce Pain, Increase Hope, and Build Meaningful Connections.* Oakland, CA: New Harbinger Publications.

Ruriani, A. 2023. *Big Feelings Survival Guide: A Creative Workbook for Mental Health.* New York: Workman Publishing Company.

Singh, A. A. 2018. *The Queer and Transgender Resilience Workbook: Skills for Navigating Sexual Orientation and Gender Expression.* Oakland, CA: New Harbinger Publications.

Walker, R. 2023. *The Unapologetic Workbook for Black Mental Health: A Step-by-Step Guide to Build Psychological Fortitude and Reclaim Wellness.* Oakland, CA: New Harbinger Publications.

Websites

The American Association of Suicidology hosts a website with information and resources for people struggling with suicidal thoughts and the people who care about them: http://suicidology.org.

The American Foundation for Suicide Prevention is an organization that provides support and information for people struggling with suicidal thoughts and people who are grieving after losing someone to suicide: http://afsp.org.

The International Association for Suicide Prevention is a global organization focused on suicide prevention. Their website is educational and provides helpful resources: http://www.iasp.info.

Suicide Prevention Resource Center is a website that compiles suicide prevention information from diverse sources: http://sprc.org.

Books for Clinicians

Bryan, C. J., and M. D. Rudd. 2018. *Brief Cognitive-Behavioral Therapy for Suicide Prevention.* New York: The Guilford Press.

Erbacher, T. A., J. B. Singer, and S. Poland. 2023. *Suicide in Schools: A Practitioner's Guide to Multi-Level Prevention, Assessment, Intervention, and Postvention*, 2nd ed. New York: Routledge.

Freedenthal, S. 2018. *Helping the Suicidal Person: Tips and Techniques for Professionals*. New York: Routledge.

Jobes, D. A. 2023. *Managing Suicidal Risk: A Collaborative Approach*, 3rd ed. New York: Guilford Press.

Joiner, T. E. 2005. *Why People Die by Suicide*. Cambridge, MA: Harvard University Press.

Joiner, T. E., K. A. Van Orden, T. K. Witte, and M. D. Rudd. 2009. *The Interpersonal Theory of Suicide: Guidance for Working with Suicidal Clients*. Washington, DC: American Psychological Association.

Linehan, M. M. 2015. *DBT Skills Training Manual*, 2nd ed. New York: Guilford Press.

O'Connor, R. 2022. *When It Is Darkest: Why People Die by Suicide and What We Can Do to Prevent It*. London: Vermilion.

ACKNOWLEDGMENTS

I'm immensely appreciative of the entire team at New Harbinger, especially Ryan Buresh, for the opportunity and shared vision of making suicide prevention strategies more accessible to all who need them, and Iris van de Pavert, for her patience and exquisite editing.

I'm grateful for every patient I've had the honor to work with; thank you for your vulnerability and openness to growth. Please know I cherished our time together and am always wishing you well. To my own therapists throughout my life, thank you; your wisdom and my memories of your caring nature show up for me at unexpected times.

I'm also deeply grateful for my graduate school mentor, Thomas Joiner, for the gifts of learning about suicide prevention, clinical psychology, and so much more from the absolute best.

To my family—including the Gordons, Robertsons, McIntyres, Martens, Dorgers, Hemmerles, Durms, Donohues, and Pronos—thank you for being such supportive, loving, and exceptionally fun people.

To my dear friends—past and present—for our connections and laughter through some of the hardest parts of life. I want to especially thank Joel Minden, Yessenia Castro, Leonardo Bobadilla, Wendy and Rob Gordon, Diane Bentley, Stacey Wicker, Ted Bender, Kim Van Orden, Tracy Witte, April Smith, and Jill Holm-Denoma.

Many thanks to my former students, current friends, and colleagues for all you have taught me—especially Brandon Saxton, Samantha Myhre, Betsy Carter, Darren Carter, Allison Perry, Mun Yee Kwan, and Valerie Douglas; I'm so proud of all of you.

And to my Equip colleagues; it's a dream and honor to work with you to make eating disorder recovery accessible for all.

REFERENCES

Bryan, C. J., and M. D. Rudd. 2018. *Brief Cognitive-Behavioral Therapy for Suicide Prevention.* New York: Guilford Press.

Bush, N. E., S. K. Dobscha, R. Crumpton, L. M. Denneson, J. E. Hoffman, A. Crain, R. Cromer, and J. Kinn. 2015. "A Virtual Hope Box Smartphone App as an Accessory to Therapy: Proof-of-Concept in a Clinical Sample of Veterans." *Suicide and Life-Threatening Behavior* 45(1): 1–9. http://doi.org/10.1111/sltb.12103.

Coopersmith, D. D. L., O. Ryan, R. G. Fortgang, A. J. Millner, E. M. Kleiman, and M. K. Nock. 2023. "Mapping the Timescale of Suicidal Thinking." *Proceedings of the National Academy of Sciences* 120(17): e2215434120. http://doi.org/10.1073/pnas.2215434120.

Denneson, L. M., D. J. Smolenski, B. W. Bauer, S. K. Dobscha, and N. E. Bush. 2019. "The Mediating Role of Coping Self-Efficacy in Hope Box Use and Suicidal Ideation Severity." *Archives of Suicide Research* 23(2): 234–246. http://doi.org/10.1080/13811118.2018.1456383.

Frankl, V. E. 1959/2006. *Man's Search for Meaning.* Boston: Beacon Press.

Holt-Lunstad, J., T. B. Smith, M. Baker, T. Harris, and D. Stephenson. 2015. "Loneliness and Social Isolation as Risk Factors for Mortality: A Meta-Analytic Review." *Perspectives on Psychological Science* 10(2): 227–237. http://doi.org/10.1177/1745691614568352.

Jobes, D. A. 2023. *Managing Suicidal Risk: A Collaborative Approach*, 3rd ed. New York: Guilford Press.

Joiner, T. E. 2005. *Why People Die by Suicide.* Cambridge, MA: Harvard University Press.

Klonsky, E. D., M. C. Pachkowski, A. Shahnaz, and A. M. May. 2021. "The Three-Step Theory of Suicide: Description, Evidence, and Some

Useful Points of Clarification." *Preventive Medicine* 152: 106549. http://doi.org/10.1016/j.ypmed.2021.106549.

Linehan, M. M. 2015. *DBT Skills Training Manual*, 2nd ed. New York: Guilford Press.

O'Connor, R. 2022. *When It Is Darkest: Why People Die by Suicide and What We Can Do to Prevent It*. London: Vermilion.

Pettit, J. W., and R. M. Hill. 2022. *Overcoming Suicidal Thoughts for Teens: CBT Activities to Reduce Pain, Increase Hope, and Build Meaningful Connections*. Oakland, CA: New Harbinger Publications.

Rogers, M. L., A. R. Gai, A. Lieberman, K. Musacchio Schafer, and T. E. Joiner. 2022. "Why Does Safety Planning Prevent Suicidal Behavior?" *Professional Psychology: Research and Practice* 53(1): 33–41. http://doi.org/10.1037/pro0000427.

Stanley, B., G. K. Brown, L. A. Brenner, H. C. Galfalvy, G. W. Currier, K. L. Knox, S. R. Chaudhury, A. L. Bush, and K. L. Green. 2018. "Comparison of the Safety Planning Intervention with Follow-Up vs. Usual Care of Suicidal Patients Treated in the Emergency Department." *JAMA Psychiatry* 75(9): 894–900. http://doi.org/10.1001/jamapsychiatry.2018.1776.

Van Orden, K. A., T. K. Witte, K. C. Cukrowicz, S. Braithwaite, E. A. Selby, and T. E. Joiner Jr. 2010. "The Interpersonal Theory of Suicide." *Psychological Review* 117(2): 575–600. http://doi.org.10.1037/a0018697.

Wenzel, A., G. K. Brown, and A. T. Beck. 2009. *Cognitive Therapy for Suicidal Patients: Scientific and Clinical Applications*. Washington, DC: American Psychological Association.

Kathryn Hope Gordon, PhD, is a licensed clinical psychologist who specializes in cognitive behavioral therapy (CBT). Gordon is also an educator who trains therapists in compassionate, scientifically informed mental health care. She was a professor for ten years, and has published more than eighty peer-reviewed articles and book chapters on suicidal behavior, disordered eating, and related topics. She is author of *The Suicidal Thoughts Workbook*.

Foreword writer **Thomas Ellis Joiner Jr., PhD**, is Bright-Burton professor of psychology, and director of the University Psychology Clinic at Florida State University. He has served as associate editor of the *Journal of Behavior Therapy*; and sits on ten editorial boards, including that of the *Journal of Consulting and Clinical Psychology*.

FROM OUR COFOUNDER—

As cofounder of New Harbinger and a clinical psychologist since 1978, I know that emotional problems are best helped with evidence-based therapies. These are the treatments derived from scientific research (randomized controlled trials) that show what works. Whether these treatments are delivered by trained clinicians or found in a self-help book, they are designed to provide you with proven strategies to overcome your problem.

Therapies that aren't evidence-based—whether offered by clinicians or in books—are much less likely to help. In fact, therapies that aren't guided by science may not help you at all. That's why this New Harbinger book is based on scientific evidence that the treatment can relieve emotional pain.

This is important: if this book isn't enough, and you need the help of a skilled therapist, use the following resources to find a clinician trained in the evidence-based protocols appropriate for your problem. And if you need more support—a community that understands what you're going through and can show you ways to cope—resources for that are provided below, as well.

Real help is available for the problems you have been struggling with. The skills you can learn from evidence-based therapies will change your life.

Matthew McKay, PhD
Cofounder, New Harbinger Publications

If you need a therapist, the following organization can help you find a therapist trained in cognitive behavioral therapy (CBT).

The Association for Behavioral & Cognitive Therapies (ABCT) Find-a-Therapist service offers a list of therapists schooled in CBT techniques. Therapists listed are licensed professionals who have met the membership requirements of ABCT and who have chosen to appear in the directory.
Please visit www.abct.org and click on Find a Therapist.

The Suicide & Crisis Lifeline
24 hours a day
If you or someone you love is dealing with a crisis right now, please call or text 988 or go to 988lifeline.org to reach the Suicide & Crisis Lifeline

For more New Harbinger books, visit www.newharbinger.com

MORE BOOKS from
NEW HARBINGER PUBLICATIONS

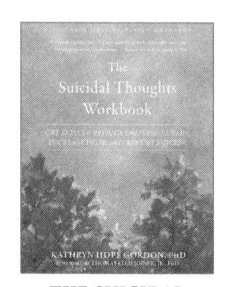

THE SUICIDAL THOUGHTS WORKBOOK
CBT Skills to Reduce Emotional Pain, Increase Hope, and Prevent Suicide
978-1684037025 / US $21.95

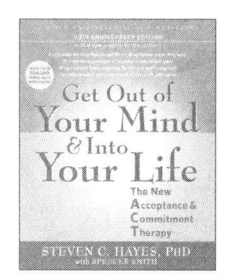

GET OUT OF YOUR MIND AND INTO YOUR LIFE
The New Acceptance and Commitment Therapy
978-1648487750 / US $24.95

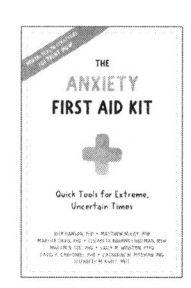

THE ANXIETY FIRST AID KIT
Quick Tools for Extreme, Uncertain Times
978-1684038480 / US $16.95

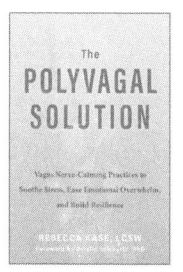

THE POLYVAGAL SOLUTION
Vagus Nerve-Calming Practices to Soothe Stress, Ease Emotional Overwhelm, and Build Resilience
978-1648484124 / US $19.95

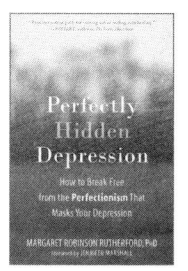

PERFECTLY HIDDEN DEPRESSION
How to Break Free from the Perfectionism That Masks Your Depression
978-1684033584 / US $21.95

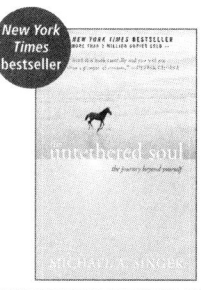

THE UNTETHERED SOUL
The Journey Beyond Yourself
978-1572245372 / US $18.95

newharbingerpublications
1-800-748-6273 / newharbinger.com
(VISA, MC, AMEX / prices subject to change without notice)   Follow Us

Don't miss out on new books from New Harbinger.
Subscribe to our email list at **newharbinger.com/subscribe**